The Workings of the Brain

The Workings of the Brain

Development, Memory, and Perception

. . .

READINGS FROM
SCIENTIFIC AMERICAN MAGAZINE

Edited by

Rodolfo R. Llinás
New York University Medical Center

W. H. FREEMAN AND COMPANY
New York

Some of the SCIENTIFIC AMERICAN articles in *The Work-ings of the Brain* are available as separate offprints. For a complete list of articles now available as Offprints, write to Product Manager, Marketing Department, W. H. Freeman and Company, 41 Madison Avenue, New York, New York 10010.

Library of Congress Cataloging-in-Publication Data

The workings of the brain.

Includes bibliographical references.

1. Brain. 2. Neurophysiology. 3. Neuropsychology.
I. Llinás, Rodolfo R. (Rodolfo Riascos), 1934–
II. Scientific American.
QP376.W84   1990   612.8'2   89-17196
ISBN 0-7167-2071-X

Printed in the United States of America

1 2 3 4 5 6 7 8 9 0   RRD   8 9

CONTENTS

SECTION IV:
OF SYMMETRY, IMAGINING AND DREAMING

SECTION V: BRAIN MODELS

Note on cross-references to SCIENTIFIC AMERICAN *articles:* Articles included in this book are referred to by chapter number and title; articles not included in this book but available as Offprints are referred to by title, date of publication and Offprint number; articles not in this book and not available as Offprints are referred to by title and date of publication.

Introduction

The trend in the study of the brain has clearly been toward analysis. We have seen, comparatively speaking, only limited attempts from a synthesis point of view. This reductionist trend is understandable: analytic tools have produced the most precise and scientifically rigorous results, not only in neurobiology but in almost every aspect of science. Indeed, in neurobiology the study of the neuronal morphology, physiology, biophysics, biochemistry and pharmacology over the past decade or so has completely changed our view of the manner in which neurons operate. (See, for example, the SCIENTIFIC AMERICAN articles in the companion volume *The Biology of the Brain: From Neurons to Networks.*)

The understanding of brain function, however, must ultimately be a synthetic effort. Two schools of thought have been slowly evolving that have defined the problem of developing such an understanding. One, which I consider to be somewhat pessimistic, suggests that as further information is gathered at different levels, a truly synthetic view of brain function will become more elusive. The other view, with which I identify, holds that understanding brain functions can ultimately be attained only through the acquisition of detailed knowledge and, further, that the scientific method allows no alternative. We can, however, encourage the latter process by designing experiments that lead toward the development of global theories of brain function, since only contextual knowledge will serve to engender complete understanding. While the ultimate synthesis is, assuredly, a long way off, first attempts to define global brain function are nevertheless worthwhile. That these early attempts will be incomplete and, in some cases, misguided there is no doubt, but progress can only occur when risks are taken.

For this volume on the workings of the brain, I have selected ten SCIENTIFIC AMERICAN articles. These represent major aspects of brain morphology and function that are now thought to be sufficiently well understood to serve as the basis for synthesis. Also represented are those areas that appear promising enough to be considered as nucleation points for the acquisition of future knowledge about the ways of the brain. Ultimately we must consider that the functions of the brain must reduce to the ability to predict future events to ensure survival. Such predictions are made on the basis of an internal image of reality manufactured in the brain by information arising from the sense organs.

Evolution and Form

In Chapter 1, ''Paleontology and the Evolution of Mind,'' Harry J. Jerison reminds us that brains have evolved at different rates, as shown by comparative studies of presently living as well as extinct vertebrates. These studies also demonstrate that the brains of different vertebrates are organized around quite different sets of operational rules. In lower vertebrates brain function operates on the basis of fixed-action patterns that only allow selection among preestablished behavioral postures, such as the fight or flight patterns seen in most animals facing danger. Jerison explains that in these animals brain development has evolved toward perfecting the fixed-action patterns that provide the most efficient sensory motor transformations possible and show a very restricted learning repertoire. Among the intermediate vertebrates, such as birds, fixed-action patterns are augmented by a plastic set of functional properties represented by a clear learning ability. In these species enriched brain function is attained by modulation and elaboration of fixed-action patterns, as exemplified by the individual variance in bird songs. In mammals a new form of brain function is attained. Rather than the further refinement of fixed-action patterns, a different approach to brain development has extended our realm of possible responses to given stimuli and enhanced our capacity for learning and memory, replacing the stereotypical brain function of lower forms. Indeed, it is the ability to formulate solutions other than the generically prescribed ones — that is, the ability to be creative — that characterizes higher nervous activity, particularly that of human beings. Thus we have the different forms of artistic expression, the development of language and the development of truly abstract thinking as it occurs, for example, in science and philosophy. Yet the relation with the evolutionary past is evident in so far as fixed-action patterns, especially those involving emotions, are clearly present in humans.

The movement away from fixed-action patterns and the qualitative difference in computation that implements this change are clearly correlated with enlarged brain size compared to body size. For example, the size of the cerebral cortex of humans has increased threefold over the past million years in comparison with that of most advanced primates. The cerebellar cortex, which mediates the coordination of movements, has actually grown four times in size during the same period. Jerison suggests that the vastly increased number of elements and connections present in the higher vertebrates result in properties that were simply not present before and, as such, are only casually related to previous stages of the evolution of the nervous system. These new properties pertain to the cognitive rather than the fixed-action sphere, that is, to the ability to know, instead of simply responding appropriately but blindly, as is the case for lower forms.

In Chapter 2, ''The Organization of the Brain,'' Walle J. H. Nauta and Michael Feirtag present an integrated view of human brain anatomy. The authors are careful to emphasize that their approach is mostly descriptive. They enter the brain and follow the different pathways, giving a unique description of where things are without dully elaborate details of their functions. The picture they present of the organization of the brain recapitulates, in a gross manner, its evolution from the more primitive patterns of sensory motor transformations residing in the spinal cord and the brain stem. It is in the latter region that the seat of autonomic brain function resides in its most primitive form, controlling the involuntary functions of respiration, swallowing, coughing, vomiting and balance. This site also governs the orientation of the body with respect to the gravitational field and the regulation of one of the most profound properties of the nervous system — the ability to be awake and aware or to sleep and be unaware of the external world. Superimposed on this autonomic set of integrated levels are the olfactory, auditory and visual systems, the so-called telereceptors, which give information to the brain about events that occur at a distance. With them comes the possibility that nuclei such as those of the thalamus and their projection to the cerebral cortex can be elaborated to give computational richness to sensory and motor functions beyond the simple transformations of sensory input to motor output. Moreover, the integration of cortical, temporal, parietal and frontal lobes through the so-called association cortices serves as a bridge between the truly analytic systems, such as the sensory system, and the executive capabilities represented by the motor centers. The motor centers, which control movement, represent the only channel of communication between the external world and the ''internal reality'' generated by brain functions.

Development and Plasticity

How do the different levels of brain complexity described above arise from a self-organizing system without prior knowledge of what its connectivity should be? The construction of complex systems from a set of predetermined instructions with a clear goal in mind is the typical methodology followed by science and engineering. That approach is totally different from the self-construction of a system that utilizes clues and rules for growth and connectivity that are not dictated by the functional properties that the neuronal circuits will ultimately serve in the developed brain. This issue is addressed in Chapter 3, "The Development of the Brain," by W. Maxwell Cowan. He indicates that the process of building a brain is one of generating distinct topographical connections, which in their earliest state are not neural but glial in origin. Such glial architecture can be considered the scaffolding neurons use in creating the neuronal circuits that ultimately characterize brain tissue. These early scaffoldings are continuously used during development. Thus as new neuronal elements appear they invade the same territory and compete for it in a manner not very different from that of animal societies.

Early in development large numbers of neurons are generated—far more than will be utilized by the adult brain. The ultimate modus operandi of the system is the selection of individual neurons in accordance with their success in establishing appropriate synaptic connections. What is truly surprising is the violent nature of this selection process and that cell suicide, not murder, is the prevailing mechanism for this population control. The ferocity of these early stages is then followed by the more subtle level of "embellished specific intercellular contact" that characterizes maturity and will last the rest of one's life. The events that guide neuronal connectivity are still a matter of dispute. Adhesiveness between neurons and the presence of specific markers and their modulation by neuronal function continue to be the most attractive candidates for the developing organization of the brain.

However, at least in lower vertebrates, the nervous system does not necessarily come to maturity and then remain at a more or less stationary level. Chapter 4, "The Development of Maps and Stripes in the Brain," by Martha Constantine-Paton and Margaret I. Law, makes an interesting and important point about the manner in which development proceeds in the frog. The optics of the front of the eye evolves to project well-focused light images onto the receptor surface of the neuronal network located in the back of the eye, known as the retina. This network is exquisitely organized spatially to accept, enhance and color-code these light images. The network in turn projects the image into the nervous system using transient electrical signals that are conducted by the optic nerve. The developmental puzzle here is the organization of the neuronal connectivity that allows a point-to-point communication between the retina and the receiving station, the optic tectum. The problem is compounded by the fact that information received by two eyes must be organized into a single image. Furthermore, the size of the frog tectum is not constant. Unlike the human brain, where the number of neurons is fixed in the first few years of life, the frog's tectum continues to grow throughout its life, as do the eyes and the optic nerve. With the enlargement of the tectum the retinal cell projections must also change, but the problem does not end there. In order to be operational the tectum must always be connected to the rest of the brain in an organized manner. Thus, in order to keep the geometric transformations that allow sensory-motor control to remain invariant despite continuous connectivity displacement, the tectal projection must also be redistributed. Based on these findings, Constantine-Paton and Law propose that, in addition to adhesiveness and the presence of chemical attractors, connectivity must also be governed by neuronal activity. Function thereby becomes another parameter in the specification of networks in the central nervous system.

We can conclude that the nervous system may be viewed as organized into a defined set of suborgans that arise out of a partly chaotic initial connectivity. This pseudochaos sorts itself out by utilizing local cues, such as the adhesiveness and chemistry of the immediate environment, without any reference to its ultimate function in the adult animal. However, even after the connectivity is attained it seems clear that function hones the properties of the connections to adapt to the environment in which the animal lives—that is, function modulates anatomy.

Emotion and Memory

Once a nervous system is developed and operational, another very important question arises: How does the brain's computational power serve the survival of the individual? It is well known in the politics of war that possession does not imply usage; similarly, possession of a particular computational ability of the brain does not demand or even assure its ultimate deployment. Other ingredients besides possession are required to activate certain functions. One important factor is referred to as *drive*. In its most primitive form drive is either positive or negative: Reward and punishment must somehow be built into the system if it is to operate at all. It has been well known by all and admitted by some that drive fuels and often rules the human mind. Indeed, as David Hume put it, our intellect is the slave of our passions.

In Chapter 5, "The Reward System of the Brain," Aryeh Routtenberg points out that the discovery of brain pleasure centers came long after the philosophical view that pain is localized in the brain. It is only recently that neuroscientists have been able to demonstrate that pleasure is a parameter in its own right. Routtenberg reviews the literature on this subject, which indicates that certain nuclei in the brain stem and hypothalamus are nodal points that, upon electrical stimulation, can generate responses congruous with pleasurable sensations. Stimulation of the anterior hypothalamus generates behavior suggesting that the animal is driven in an insatiable manner. For example, when presented with a lever that triggers such stimulation, the animal will press the lever as fast as possible and without respite. This is probably the type of neuronal activity that is behind pure drive. The pleasure obtained by the drive toward a goal is a distinct state that fuels the process itself.

The second area of self-stimulation, located in the posterior lateral hypothalamus, generates an altogether different pattern of behavior. The animal presses the lever at a more leisurely pace and produces a stereotypical behavior after every activation of the lever, suggesting a modicum of satiation. After every movement of the lever, a rat, for example, may move its head back and open its mouth, a movement that in humans would indicate a clear pleasure sensation.

In short, the anterior hypothalamus seems to produce blind drive, without satiation or reward other than by its continuation. The second form of pleasure response seems to build to a peak and produce a degree of satiation. Clearly, both forms of pleasure response are required—one to get there, the other to enjoy having gotten there. Our understanding of these systems is far from complete. The whole issue of motivation is still in its most primitive level of explanation. Nevertheless, these systems clearly will be implicated in many psychiatric disorders and in the use of so-called recreational drugs. Such drugs obviously tap directly into these circuits and, by circumventing normal pathways, give the recipients pleasure without requiring any labor in its attainment.

One of the elements that characterizes higher brain function most clearly is the acquisition of memory. The different types of memory and the neurological machinery that embodies them are presented in general form in Chapter 6, "The Anatomy of Memory," by Mortimer Mishkin and Tim Appenzeller. Here the relevant brain systems include the cortical analyzers, the associated cortex, the paleocortex (hippocampus), their interconnections and, especially, the well-defined network known as the limbic system. Mishkin and Appenzeller describe (on the basis of work on humans and monkeys) the brain areas most directly related to learning and remembering, in particular, the importance of the hippocampus in the consolidation of memory. Bilateral lesion of the hippocampus produces the inability to acquire new knowledge, but does not eradicate prior knowledge. This clearly indicates that the hippocampus is required for the acquisition but not for the retention of memories, the latter being a more distinct property. Indeed, while the inability to acquire new memories is always considered when damage of the hippocampus occurs, the capacity of recollection may be equally at fault. Unfortunately, because of this overlap it is difficult to address memory storage without testing recall.

Of Symmetry, Imagining and Dreaming

Returning to the brain as a whole, there is one basic question that has been asked for a very long time: What are the differences between the two cerebral hemispheres? That the right and left hemispheres differ anatomically in most people and that they have different functions is the subject of Chapter 7, "Specializations of the Human Brain," by Norman Geschwind. The anatomical differences, as in the thickness of a particular part of the cortex or its total weight, can be compared to the differences between human faces and are not extraordinary. By contrast, the functional deficits that follow lesions of corresponding regions in one or the other hemisphere may be strikingly different. The area that controls the premotor articulation of speech, known as Broca's area, is located for right-handed people in the left hemisphere in front and below the area known as the motor cortex, which controls the execution initiation of movement. Lesions of Broca's area produce impairment of speech, but a lesion of the symmetrical counterpart on the right side produces no great loss in the ability to speak. A similar set of examples may be encountered for other brain functions where specialization of function is lateralized.

Interestingly enough, such lateralization may be found in primates and songbirds. The lesson to be learned from these observations is that the brain is composed of quite specialized systems; not all parts of the cortex are equipotential. In short, the two hemispheres are specialized for different functions. One of the most exciting issues raised by this type of study is the reason for such specialization. Other functions, on the other hand, are not strongly lateralized. Thus bilateral damage of the hippocampus produces the inability to acquire new knowledge but unilateral damage does not. A similar observation may be made regarding the ability to recognize faces, which also is only lost following a bilateral lesion. The most general conclusion seems to be that particular neuronal circuits having a given connectivity will be capable of doing certain tasks in a more efficient manner than other circuits, that is, a certain amount of hardware specialization is required for different functions. Therefore, the brain is not a universal computing machine, but a more specialized system of computation.

Whether scientific methodology of any type might ultimately be able to address subjective experience in an unambiguous manner has been an open question until rather recently. The reason for such doubt is related to the belief that purely subjective experience cannot be grasped by an objective methodology. Yet, in an extraordinarily elegant set of experiments Lynn A. Cooper and Roger N. Shepard have attempted to measure directly the functional properties of a subjective mental process, which are discussed in Chapter 8, "Turning Something Over in the Mind." The question they posed was when imagining a rotating object, is there any way for an external observer to determine the speed and direction with which the imaginary object is rotating in the subject's imagination. The experiments consisted of allowing individuals to observe computer-generated images resembling armlike structures made of cubes. The subjects were then given a second picture of the same object rotated by a certain number of degrees to the right or left. The time between the presentation of the second picture and its recognition by the subject indicated that mental rotation proceeded at an average angular speed of 35 degrees per second. The authors also demonstrated that if the rotation was restricted to two dimensions, the subject's computational time was not much shorter. These experiments suggest that internal representation tends to reproduce not only the shapes of objects in the external world, but also the dynamic components of objects in motion. In other words, the thinking process may recreate some of the external properties of objects in physical space and may require the computation of intermediate stages in order to arrive at the final position of an image.

Another investigation that alerts us to the possibility of objective measurement of basically intrinsic states is the study of dreaming without paralysis. It has been known for many years that during dreaming states animals and humans demonstrate a total muscular paralysis. This paralysis prevents us from responding physically to our dreams and, therefore, our oneiric confabulations may rage in the reassurance of total peripheral discretion. Such reassurance is clearly vital to the survival of the individual, who may otherwise respond to imaginary events with violent movements. Such behavior, totally unguided by perception, could easily result in injury to oneself or to one's bedpartner. Adrian R. Morrison alludes in Chapter 9, "A Window on the Sleeping Brain," to the fact that following localized lesions in the brainstem, the paralysis that usually accompanies sleep may no longer occur and the individual will act out his dreams. It may be possible to witness the workings of the brain in the absence of self-criticism and restraint by disconnecting this inhibitory action on the motor system. What this paradigm may teach us about the nature of dreaming needs to be explored.

Brain Models

Last is the issue of whether the properties that we consider to be the exclusive domain of brain function—coordinated movement, understanding or generating language, thinking and feeling—are in fact biological properties. If they are not they must be computational properties. This statement may be initially difficult to understand, but there are wonderful examples of similar queries from other periods in history. In the 13th and 14th centuries scholars agreed that flight must be a biological property since only living systems were capable of controlled flight. To these scholars the only route to an understanding of flight was through study of the biology of flight, such as the study of feathers. Yet to Leonardo da Vinci it seems to have been clear that flight was not a biological property but rather an aerodynamic property that can be embedded in a biological or nonbiological framework. Similarly, we may conceive of intelligence or feeling as "computational" properties that may, in principle, be embodied in any system capable of supporting such a computational load. Whether such views will ultimately be proven correct cannot be foretold, but artificial computational systems are becoming sufficiently intricate for us to be confident that such a question may be answered in the not-too-distant future. Perhaps the most exciting development over the past five years in this respect has been the advent of connectivism, a child of both artificial intelligence and the neurosciences.

Chapter 10, "Collective Computation in Neuron-like Circuits," by David W. Tank and John J. Hopfield is an excellent example of the types of modeling and ideas that are presently being developed in the study of neural networks. The models developed so far are most syntactical in character — that

is, they model the ability of a particular device to translate one set of instructions into a different format, such as transforming written into spoken language but without an understanding of that which is read or spoken. Some believe, however, that such devices may also be capable of semantics, in the sense of setting information into context. In any event, two important results are likely to follow from this effort: the development of a set of intelligent devices and the attainment of an heuristic tool that would allow us to understand brain functions. It is possible that many of the most intransigent questions about the mind may simply melt away as we better understand the computational properties of large ensembles of elements working in parallel, for that is what appears to characterize the machinery of the brain.

Rodolfo R. Llinás

The Workings of the Brain

SECTION

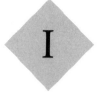

I

EVOLUTION AND FORM

· · ·

Paleoneurology and the Evolution of Mind

Tracing changes in the relation between brain size and body size in various groups of fossil and contemporary animals sheds light not only on the evolution but also on the nature of intelligence.

· · ·

Harry J. Jerison
January, 1976

The mind evolved. Paleoneurology, which deals with the evidence of nervous systems in fossil animals, provides new clues to the nature of that evolution. Integrated with information about the variety of brains and behaviors in living vertebrates and knowledge of how neural tissue is packaged in brains, the fossil record can be interpreted to develop a coherent account of the evolution of intelligence over the 500-million-year span of vertebrate history. That account provides fresh perspectives on the nature of intelligence as a biological phenomenon.

The approach complements more traditional ways of studying the evolution of mind: ethological analyses, based on naturalistic observations of species-typical behaviors of living animals, and psychological studies, which measure the competence of various species in standardized laboratory tests. The traditional analyses build on evolutionary relations among living animals to reconstruct the evolution of behaviors; the variety of present patterns of behavior are projected backward in time to probable ancestral patterns. With paleoneurological data, on the other hand, the approach to the evolutionary history of the brain is direct, and the history is interpreted in the light of present-day relations between brain and behavior.

The strategy of the paleoneurological analysis of mind is to identify a morphological trait as a correlate of mind, or biological intelligence. If the mind evolved, certain trends in the evolution of that correlated trait should be evident in the fossil record. For example, since there are obviously different grades in the distribution of intelligence or mind in living animals, it should be possible to measure an increase and a diversification of the morphological trait in successive geological periods.

Charles Darwin was the author of an early statement of one hypothesis that relates mind to morphology when he wrote in *The Descent of Man*: "No one, I presume, doubts that the large proportion which the size of man's brain bears to his body, compared to the same proportion in the gorilla or orang, is closely connected with is mental powers." Some 80 years later Karl Spencer Lashley's more careful and explicit statement of the hypothesis made it applicable to the analysis of morphological data: "The only neurological character for which a correlation with behavioral capacity in different animals is supported by significant evidence is the total mass of tissue, or rather, the index of cephalization . . . which seems to represent the amount of brain tissue in excess of that required for transmitting impulses to and from the integrative centers."

The index, a measure of relative brain size, is defined as total brain size divided by the two-thirds power of the body size. (The exponent has to do with the relation between surface and volume, as I shall explain further along.) The ratio can be visualized if one plots data reflecting the present diversity of brain and body sizes in vertebrates (see Figure

1.1). Lashley's statement is borne out by the clear differentiation between "lower" and "higher" vertebrates and by the fact that the arrays of points representing both groups are similarly oriented at a slope of ⅔. It is easy to imagine the higher vertebrates as having evolved from a lower vertebrate grade as the result of the vertical displacement of a set of points in brain:body space. That displacement is in effect what is measured by the index of cephalization. This implies that brain size is determined by a "body-size factor" and an "encephalization factor." Lashley's hypothesis was that only the encephalization factor was involved in the evolution of mind. Birds and mammals are "higher" vertebrates because they are more highly encephalized

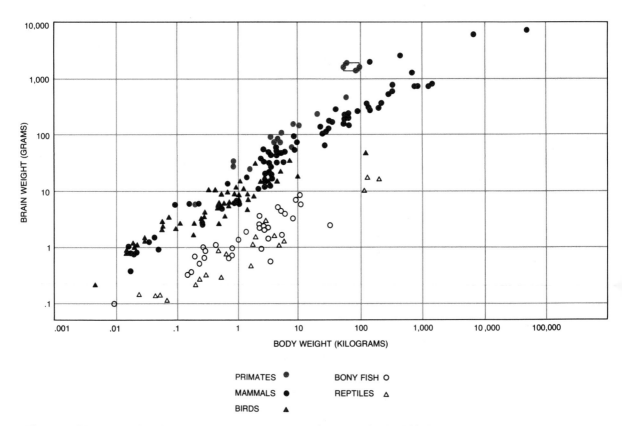

Figure 1.1 BRAIN WEIGHT is plotted against body weight for some 200 species of living vertebrates. The data were collected by George W. Crile and Daniel P. Quiring some years ago. The four colored points connected by a rectangle represent the extreme measurements reported for man, indicating that variation within a species does not loom large in comparison to the distinctions among species. Data fall into two clearly delimited groups, which may be considered to be the lower and the higher vertebrates. In both cases the data fall along a line with a slope of 2/3 on log-log coordinates: brain weight varies with the 2/3 power (which is the cube root of the square) of body weight.

and are higher on a scale of biological intelligence than reptiles and other "lower" vertebrates. That is an interpretation of the data that agrees nicely with our intuition.

To assemble paleoneurological evidence one needs to know the brain and body size of fossil vertebrates. The brain size is determined from the volume of endocranial casts, or endocasts (see Figure 1.2), that are replicas of the cranial cavity. In some cases natural endocasts are found: mineralized remains of sand or other deposits that replaced the soft tissue in a fossil skull. In other cases the fossil skull serves as the mold for a man-made acrylic or plaster endocast. The body size of the fossil vertebrate can be measured or estimated from models based on skeletal reconstructions. To take one example, the Eocene ungulate (hoofed mammal) *Uintatherium anceps* (see Figure 1.3) weighed about 1,250 kilograms; its endocast indicates a brain weight of about 290 grams. By assembling and plotting a large body of data of this kind it is possible to derive "brain : body maps," minimum convex polygons that enclose a set of brain : body points and enable one to analyze major shifts in encephalization without numerical analyses or indexes.

In Figure 1.4 a polygon for living mammals defines the region in brain : body space associated with the present mammalian grade of encephalization. The brain : body data of early fossil mammals are shown in the archaic-mammalian polygon. ("Archaic" designates taxonomic orders that are now extinct, having been replaced in their ecological niches by species from "progressive" orders.) The geologic time of the map for archaic mammals extends from the upper Jurassic period represented by the earliest well-preserved mammalian endocast (*Triconodon mordax*) to the late Eocene epoch with forms such as *Uintatherium*, or a time span of from about 150 to 40 million years ago. The polygon indicates that a single archaic mammalian grade persisted for the entire period. In the reptilian polygon the fossil data on dinosaurs, pterosaurs (flying reptiles) and therapsids (mammal-like reptiles) are entered along with the sample of living reptiles. Two fossil amphibians and one fossil fish are included, so that the reptilian polygon is a reasonable picture of the original lower grade of brain : body relations in jawed vertebrate species, the grade from which birds and mammals advanced when they first evolved.

The brain : body maps lead to a number of interesting conclusions:

1. Living reptiles have not departed significantly from their ancestral condition. A single brain : body map includes all the fossil and living species for which we have data, showing that the adaptive radiation of the reptiles and other lower vertebrates was accomplished without any major advances in relative brain size.

2. Adding fossil reptiles extends the reptilian polygon while maintaining its orientation in brain : body space. This fact and the data on mammals suggest that a fundamental biological process determines the orientation at a slope of about $2/3$. Because the coordinate system is logarithmic the slope can be interpreted as providing exponents for the measures of body and brain (2 for the square units of a body surface and 3 for the cubic units of a brain volume) and thus for the exponent of $2/3$ in the index of cephalization. That is a straightforward application of principles of physics. It makes sense biologically because of the way sensory and motor "surfaces" of the body are projected on the many structures that add up to the volume of the brain; maps of the cerebral cortex of mammals are often presented as grossly distorted but recognizable body surfaces drawn on a diagram of the brain.

3. Dinosaurs were not unusually "small-brained." The 10 dinosaurs that contributed data on fossil reptiles were the source of the inference about the stability of the reptilian, or lower vertebrate, condition and the uniformity of slope for both fossil reptiles and living ones. The 10 dinosaurs were clearly normal reptiles with respect to brain size.

4. Encephalization and the evolution of intelligence occurred independently in birds and in mammals, which evolved independently from two different subclasses of reptiles. (The record on fossil birds is not considered in detail in this chapter; the 150-million-year-old fossil *Archaeopteryx*, the earliest-known bird, was intermediate between the reptilian grade and the grade of living birds.)

5. The reptilian map and the two mammalian maps are similarly oriented with a slope of about $2/3$, and there are vertical displacements that indicate the progressive encephalization of the mammals.

6. Although the step from reptiles to mammals required a certain amount of encephalization (approximately a four-fold increase in relative brain size to transform a reptilian polygon into an archaic mammalian polygon), mammalian encephalization did not progress immediately but remained at a

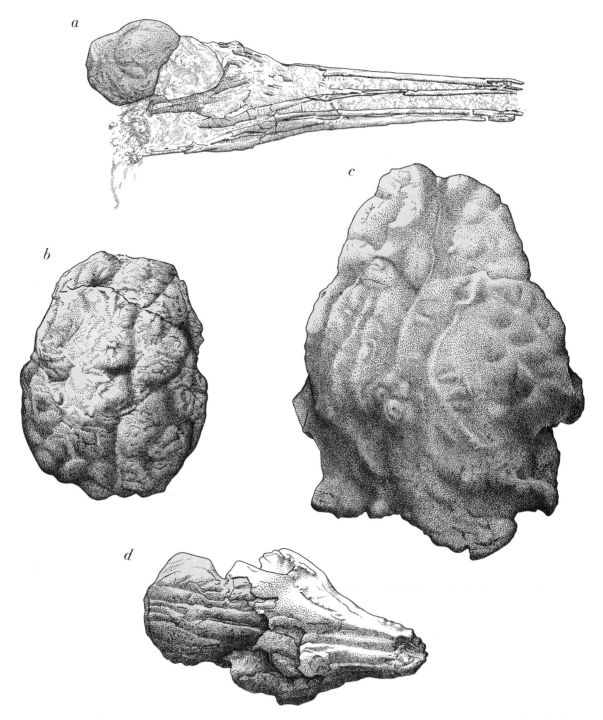

Figure 1.2 ENDOCASTS, casts of the inside of the cranial cavity, are displayed for four fossil animals. These endocasts, each drawn about one and a quarter times actual size, are natural ones: mineralized remains of sand or other deposits that replaced the soft tissues in the fossil skulls. The endocast of *Numenius gypsorum*, a bird of the Eocene (about 40 million years ago), is still in place in the long-beaked skull (*a*). The endocasts removed from their craniums are of *Potamotherium* (*b*), an otterlike Oligocene carnivore (about 25 million years ago), and *Dicrocerus* (*c*), an ungulate, or hoofed herbivore, from the Miocene (15 million years ago). The endocast of *Cainotherium* (*d*), an Oligocene ungulate, has parts of the skull in place. Casts are from the Muséum d'Histoire Naturelle in Paris.

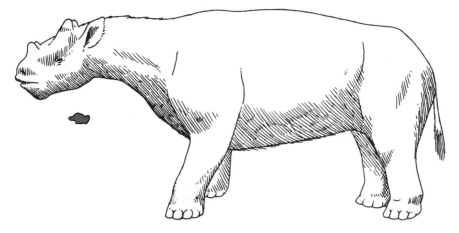

Figure 1.3 FOSSIL ANIMALS are reconstructed on the basis of their skeletal remains in order to provide an estimate of body size to compare with the brain size derived from an endocast. The body can actually be modeled and the model's volume can be determined, or the size can be estimated from a drawing. This animal is *Uintacherium anceps*, an archaic ungulate of some 50 million years ago. It weighed about 1,250 kilograms and its brain (*color*) weighed about 290 grams. Data are plotted as point No. 12 in Figure 1.4.

steady level for at least 100 million years. The earliest and the latest of the archaic species of mammals were all at about the same grade of relative brain size, enclosed within a single rather narrow polygon. That stability for such a long period of time suggests a successful response to the selection pressures of a stable new ecological niche.

7. Progressive evolution of encephalization within the mammals came late in their history, in the last 50 million years of a time span of about 200 million years. That evolution transformed the archaic mammalian map into the map of living mammals by another four- or fivefold increase in relative brain size for the average mammal.

The final steps in encephalization are revealed in the fossil record of mammalian endocasts of the present geological era: the Cenozoic, which began approximately 65 millon years ago. Those steps are best measured with a modern version of the index of cephalization: the encephalization quotient (E.Q.), which is the actual size of the brain divided by its expected size for an average living mammal (see Figure 1.5). The expected size is determined by an equation, which states that the brain size equals the ⅔ power of the body size multiplied by a constant (.12) that represents the index of cephalization for an average living mammal.

In order to analyze the progressive evolution of encephalization in the mammals, I have computed average E.Q.'s and standard deviations for samples of fossil and living ungulates and carnivores and plotted them as a set of normal curves (see Figure 1.6) The curves have equal areas and can therefore be treated as normal probability distributions, that is, each curve shows the probability of the presence of species of the indicated degrees of encephalization in each assemblage. There was evidently a steady advance in average E.Q. during the Tertiary period (from about 65 million to about three million years ago), and there was also a diversification of E.Q that was more or less proportional to the average E.Q. Significantly, the distributions overlap in the lower range of encephalization, indicating that some relatively small-brained species persisted in all the fossil groups and that they still persist among living mammals.

These are results that one would expect if encephalization (and intelligence) evolved as other traits have. Evolution involves morphological and behavioral adaptations to a variety of niches and to the invasion of new niches. The adaptive zones occupied by successive species of carnivores and ungulates during the Tertiary period must have included many niches in which there were selective advantages for species further encephalized. As more of these niches were invaded there would have been diversification, which would in turn have affected

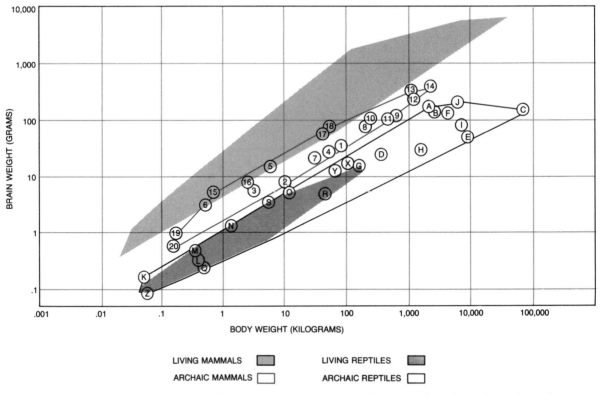

Figure 1.4 BRAIN: BODY MAPS are the minimum convex polygons that can be drawn to enclose a set of points representing brain size plotted against body size. Here the data for living mammals and reptiles have been taken from Figure 1.1. Numbered points are for archaic ungulates and carnivores; oldest is *Triconodon* (20). Fossil reptiles are dinosaurs (*A—J*), pterosaurs (*K—O*) and mammal-like reptiles (*Q—S*); two amphibians (*X, Y*) and a fish (*Z*) are included.

the frequency distributions of E.Q.'s (see Figure 1.7).

The gradual change in encephalization throughout the Tertiary period has thus far been demonstrated only for the ungulates and carnivores among the orders of mammals. Although that may be owing simply to a lack of enough data on other orders, the limited evidence on other mammals suggests a different pattern of evolution: When an adaptive zone was entered, the succession of species in that zone attained a particular grade of encephalization rapidly and then maintained it. For example, the earliest-known insectivore endocasts, from about 35 to 40 million years ago, were already at the same grade of encephalization as average living species of insectivores, namely somewhat above the

archaic level. Similarly, endocasts and body sizes for "dolphins" of about 18 million years ago, the earliest in this group of cetaceans, show that they had already reached the E.Q. level of comparable living species such as the harbor porpoise. Dolphins, as large-brained mammals, may therefore represent an evolutionary picture very different from the more or less equally encephalized human species. As we shall see, the evolution of the hominid brain to its present size is a relatively recent phenomenon, having been completed only within the past million years.

The fossil evidence on the primate brain is not as complete as that for carnivores and ungulates, but it is orderly and involves several striking fea-

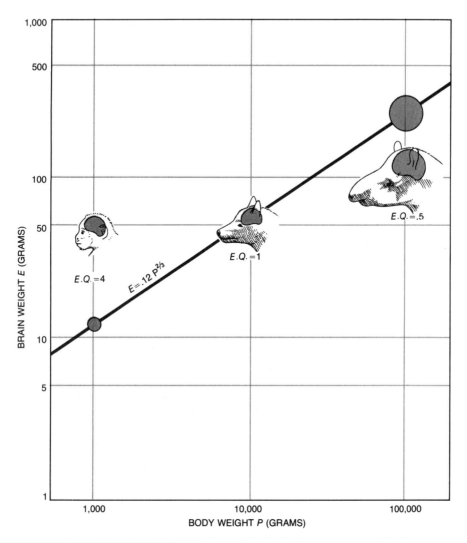

Figure 1.5 ENCEPHALIZATION QUOTIENT (E.Q.) is the ratio of an animal's actual brain size to its "expected" brain size. The expected sizes, represented by the diagonal, are given by an equation: brain size (E) equals .12 (the index of cephalization for an average mammal) times the 2/3 power of the body size (P). A hypothetical "smart" monkey has a brain four times as large (48 grams) as the expected size (12 grams) for its body size; its E.Q. is said to be 4. An "average" dog has an E.Q. of 1 and a "stupid" tapirlike animal has an E.Q. of .5.

tures. The primates have always been large-brained mammals. Early Tertiary prosimians had values of E.Q. ranging from .55 to 1.75. This can be contrasted with the range for all other early Tertiary progressive land mammals on which I have data, which is from .19 to .92. Living monkeys and apes are about twice as encephalized as other living land mammals (a mean E.Q. of 2.1 for simians as compared with 1.0 for average mammals). Primates of about 50 million years ago were also about twice as encephalized as their land-mammal contemporaries.

Encephalization within the hominids is measurable by cranial capacity rather than E.Q. (The comparison of cranial capacities is equivalent to the analysis of encephalization in species that are similar in body size, since it amounts to scaling vertically in brain : body space.) An australopithecine grade—

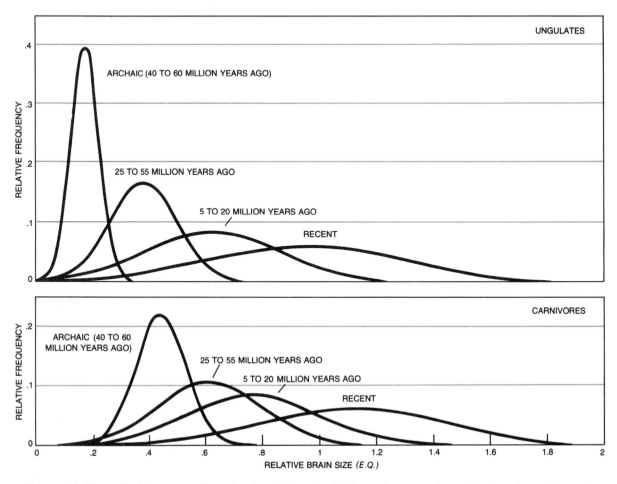

Figure 1.6 CHANGING DISTRIBUTIONS of relative brain size (E.Q.) are plotted for ungulates (*top*) and carnivores (*bottom*). Each curve gives the distribution of brain sizes for various species during specified periods; recent species are those living today. There is a steady increase in brain size and a concomitant diversification, with small-brained species persisting, shown by the flattening of successive curves. Note that these are "between species" curves. Differences within a species are usually not reflected in behavior.

a volume of about 500 milliliters—had been achieved in the early Pleistocene epoch, two or three million years ago, and probably as early as the Pliocene, five million years or more ago. A pithecanthropine grade has been recorded in a unique 800-milliliter endocast from Lake Rudolph in Kenya that is almost three million years old; the better-known true pithecanthropines are about a million years old and their cranial capacities range from about 750 to 1,250 milliliters [see "The Casts of Fossil Hominid Brains," by Ralph L. Holloway; Scientific American, July, 1974].

The earliest endocast for *Homo sapiens* is about 250,000 years old, and man's present cranial capacity ranges from about 1,000 to 2,000 milliliters. The important evolutionary fact is the rapidity and recency of the increase in encephalization in the hominid lineage. There is no evidence of a change in encephalization in any other mammals in the past five million years (see Figure 1.8). In the remainder of this article I shall discuss some critical events in the history of the vertebrates that provide clues to the causes of encephalization and also to the nature of biological intelligence.

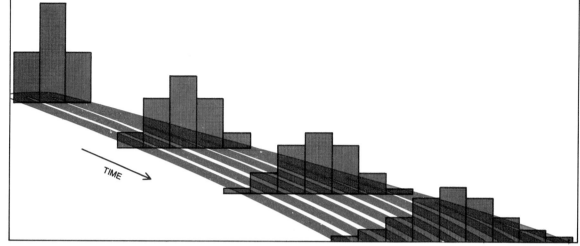

Figure 1.7 DIVERSIFICATION IN BRAIN SIZE reflects an adaptive radiation with respect to encephalization. The diverging pathways (*color*) suggest the increasing number of ecological niches making diverse demands on the brain. Niches appeared that required more encephalization, and other niches were preserved that made smaller demands. Animals adapted to a wider range of "encephalization niches" were able to survive. The bars reflect schematically the fact that distribution depends on discrete numbers of niches.

Vertebrates do not live by brains alone. That is the message from the insignificant encephalization in the many successful species of lower vertebrates and from the stability of relative brain size in the archaic mammals for at least 100 million years. The advance from fish to amphibian about 350 million years ago illustrates the conservatism in brain evolution. Here was an invasion of terrestrial niches, possibly the most demanding new adaptive zone in vertebrate history, yet according to the paleoneurological evidence there was no increase in encephalization. That was possible because the earliest amphibian required only minor alterations in the patterns of neurological and behavioral organization of its immediate ancestor among the bony fish. Sir James Gray has shown that even the adaptations for movements on land could be "conservative." The legs of an amphibian served the same function as the inertial force of water for a swimming animal, providing a fulcrum that enabled early amphibians to be little more than fish that swam on land.

In the same sense, I believe, the earliest mammals were probably only slightly modified from their reptilian predecessors: they were "reptiles" that were active at night. This view, which explains the evolution of enlarged brains in early mammals, is consistent with the general evolutionary history of reptiles of the late Paleozoic and early Mesozoic eras, about 250 million years ago. The mammal-like reptiles called therapsids were the dominant forms during the late Paleozoic era, and they were replaced during the early Mesozoic by the ruling reptiles, notably the dinosaurs. The dinosaurs and therapsids were clearly in a kind of competition for the normal niches of land reptiles, and the mammal-like reptiles lost the competition, becoming completely extinct by the mid-Mesozoic era, about 150 million years ago. The niches for which the therapsids competed and lost were for large diurnal animals that used vision as the normal sense for receiving information about events at a distance. The earliest mammals were a persistent remnant of only slightly modified therapsids, and they survived as small, nocturnal animals. They had improved auditory and olfactory systems and their visual systems were modified, with rod cells taking the place of cone cells. Both changes were appropriate for animals that were active at night.

The evolution of hearing and smell to supplement

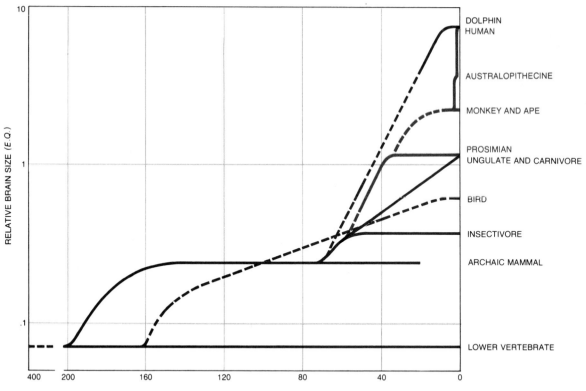

Figure 1.8 RATE OF EVOLUTION of grade of encephalization varied in different vertebrate groups and at different times. There was actually variability of brain size within groups too, so that the curves are somewhat arbitrary. In the case of cetaceans the highest grade attained is plotted to emphasize that the cetaceans that reached the dolphin grade did so long before the primates reached even an australopithecine grade; the recent and rapid evolution of the hominid brain is notable. The broken lines indicate gaps in data.

vision as a distance sense is sufficient reason for the evolution of an enlarged brain in the earliest mammals. The reason is to be found in the way neural elements are packaged in vertebrate sensory systems. In the visual system many of the circuits are in the retina, which contains an extensive and complex neural network that allows elaborate analysis of visual information. The corresponding neural elements of the auditory and olfactory systems of living vertebrates are in the brain proper (see Figure 1.9).

In the quantitative terms the effect of different modes of packaging is enormous. A small, highly visual lizard such as the American chameleon *Anolis* has in its retina at least a million sensory cells (cones) and about 100,000 ganglion cells, where the fibers of the optic nerve originate. Still other retinal neurons are involved in higher-order processing in that lizard's retina, and they must be almost as numerous as the sensory cells. The ear of *Anolis*, on the other hand, has only a few hundred sensory cells and other neural elements external to the brain. An auditory system analogous to the visual system would presumably have to have about as much integrative circuitry as there is in the retina, so that an "auditory" animal the size of *Anolis* would need space for almost a million integrative neurons and their dendritic fields to analyze inputs from the ears. There is no space for these in the middle and inner ears; the obvious place to package the additional material is in the brain itself, and solving the packaging problem would therefore require the enlargement of parts of the brain involved in audition. A similar argument would apply to an "olfactory"

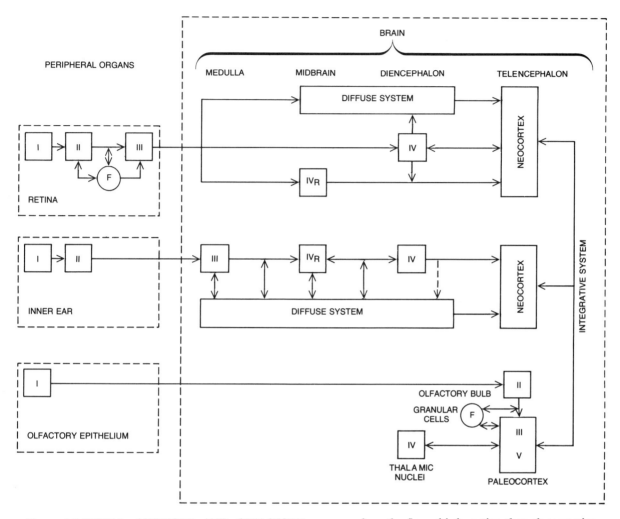

Figure 1.9 VISUAL, AUDITORY AND OLFACTORY SYSTEMS of living mammals are diagrammed in simplified schematic form to show that a much more significant fraction of the visual system than of the other two systems is packaged not in the brain but in a peripheral organ. The arrows show the flow of information through successive orders of nerve cells (*I through V*); stages labeled *IV$_R$* are parts of reflex control systems; *F* marks feedback loops. The integrative neocortical system (*right*) is specifically mammalian.

animal: its increased dependence on the sense of smell would require expansion of the forebrain systems that contain the integrative neurons of the olfactory system.

The brain of an early mammal with the body size of *Anolis* would have handled distance information in a reptilian way but with audition and olfaction as the receptor systems in place of daylight vision. Such a mammal's brain would have had to be enlarged compared with a normal Mesozoic reptilian brain in order to have space for the new neural networks that evolved to analyze nonvisual information. And so we see that the first expansion of the vertebrate brain may have been primarily a solution of a packaging problem and that it may only incidentally have resulted in the evolution of intelligence. Let us see how this crucial incidental result might have been attained.

The introduction of encephalized and finely discriminative audition and olfaction demands new ways of encoding neural information. Visual information is encoded at a retinal level with a structurally determined spatial code: the optics of the eye and the arrangement of retinal elements provide a grid that labels the location of stimulated cells. No such code is possible for sound or odors. It is difficult for us, the least olfactory of land mammals, to imagine how spatial information could be encoded with the olfactory system, but consider how such coding is accomplished by the auditory system. Animals that use echolocation to identify the source and shape of distant objects do it by translating spatial information into a temporal code. Some such localization of environmental sounds in space must have been accomplished by the early mammals if audition was for them a precise distance sense. In the evolution and functioning of the neural apparatus necessary for such behavior two dimensions of sensory experience had to be encoded by the brain: space and time.

More was needed. Imagine an early mammal coping with life at twilight, sensing stimuli from distant sources. The stimuli are recorded by reptile-like vision (modified toward the mammalian retina with rod cells for night vision), mammalian hearing and mammalian smell, all providing information from the same environmental source. It would obviously be adaptive if the information received from the different sense modalities were given a common code, or label. The integrating code would work, in all likelihood, by the labeling of stimuli in the different modalities as coming from the same object in space at a particular time. And so we have the basic constructs of human conscious experience: objects in space and time. The conscious experience is essentially a construction of nervous systems for handling incoming information in a simple, consistent way.

This leads me to a few simple propositions. Reality, or the real world we know intuitively, is a creation of the nervous system: a model of a possible world, which enables the nervous system to handle the enormous amount of information it receives and processes. (That view is similar to one presented by the English psychologist K. J. W. Craik on the nature of explanation.) The "true" or "real" world is specific to a species and is dependent on how the brain of the species works; this is as true for our own world—the world as we know it—as it is for the world of any species. (That view was made familiar by the German biologist Jakob Johann von Uexküll, who described the "perceptual worlds" of animals

and men.) The work of the brain is to create a model of a possible world rather than to record and transmit to the mind a world that is metaphysically true.

Biological intelligence, then, is a measure of the quality of the particular real world created by the brain of a particular species. The world as we know it ourselves, with the self as perhaps its most complex object, represents the human grade of biological intelligence. Different worlds are presumably constructed by different species. A very simple construction of a world may be characteristic of the lower vertebrates. As a matter of fact, no transformation of neural information—no construction—at all may be required in the lower vertebrates. Their behavior is tightly bound to specific stimuli by fixed-action patterns of response, in contrast to an "intelligence" system in which varied patterns of stimuli are transformed into invariant objects. The birds seem to be a special case. In birds the fixed-action pattern is the typical behavioral mode, and biological intelligence may be a little-used capacity. Yet experimental procedures showing that birds are well within the mammalian range of competence in performing standardized—albeit "unnatural"—learning tasks seem to affirm the basic validity of the judgment, based on relative brain size, that birds and mammals are at comparable grades of biological intelligence. Intelligence, in biological perspective, is clearly only one of several dimensions of behavior and is not the most important one for birds.

The further encephalization of the mammals beyond the archaic level involved new and peculiarly mammalian adaptations to niches that became available as a result of the extinction of dinosaurs and other ruling reptiles. These were daytime niches, and the mammalian response to them occurred in two stages. The first stage was an adaptive radiation that did not involve encephalization, in which effects were toward increases in body size; this was the archaic mammalian radiation. The second stage was a response to the new availability of daytime niches. It was inevitable that the visual system would evolve in some mammalian species and that those species would be at an adaptive advantage in daytime.

The new mammalian visual system would not be a simple retrogression to reptilian vision. Mammals had by then lost many of the reptilian visual adaptations; their normal vision was nocturnal, based on a new system of receptors (rod cells rather than cone cells) and a different analysis of the information from the receptors. Their vision must also have been much more encephalized than reptilian vision if it needed to be integrated with auditory and olfactory information. Lost adaptations do not reappear, and it is clear from the record of the mammals that their daytime vision was based on mechanisms different from those of reptiles. Mammalian vision is represented at forebrain levels, in the thalamus and the cortex, whereas reptilian vision has its most significant central representation at the level of the midbrain and is accomplished to a great extent at a retinal level.

What was the nature of the encephalized daylight visual system in progressive Tertiary mammals? A conservative approach would assume that such a system would be modeled after the other encephalized systems of the brain — the auditory, olfactory and night-vision systems — and would therefore involve the temporal encoding of spatial information and also object formation. Because the peripheral information would already have been encoded spatially, the temporal code might result in the creation of "mental images," or memories of objects and of their spatial location. That construction would also involve other sense modalities, and so integrative systems for associating information contributed by the various sense modalities would have to be expanded. That called for still further morphological encephalization.

The step to man can be analyzed in a similar way. Several unusual selection pressures may help to explain the peculiar hominid adaptations and encephalization. It is currently accepted that the early hominids were nonarboreal primates that had invaded a niche comparable to that of predatory carnivores and that they had become modified for life in such a niche. What special problems may have faced such progressive primates, assuming that, like their living relatives, they were noisy social animals with reduced olfactory systems? Their geographic range would have been considerably more extensive than that of any other living primate, and they would have had to cope with that range with a much diminished sense of smell. Olfactory labels, with which wide-ranging social carnivores such as wolves mark a territory and map a perceptual world, would not have been available to the hominids. The development of adequate labels to mark the range may have required the further develop-

ment of auditory, visual and particularly vocal capacities — the last of these acknowledging the fact that primates are noisy animals. Such a development is consistent with the evolutionary model used to analyze encephalization in other mammals. In the case of the primates it suggests the evolution of primitive language as a further solution to the problem of creating a real world that provides an adequate model for the sensory events encountered during an animal's life.

A primary model of that type postulates language as a sensory-perceptual development. The availability of vocal labels can obviously result in the capacity to communicate linguistically, but I prefer to separate the role of language in perceptual activity from its role in communication; this makes it much easier to justify the evolution of language. If there were selection pressures toward the development of language specifically for communication, we would expect the evolutionary response to be the development of "prewired" language systems with conventional sounds and symbols. Those are the typical approaches to communication in other vertebrates, and they are accomplished (as in birds) with little or no learning and with relatively small neural systems. The very flexibility and plasticity of the language systems of the human brain argue for their evolution as having been analogous to that of other sensory integrative systems, which are now known to be unusually plastic, or modifiable by early experience. (Benjamin Lee Whorf and Edward Sapir pointed out many years ago one of the maladaptive features of this flexibility of the language system, which enables different societies to develop different languages and hence different realities, often with catastrophic effects on the interactions of human communities.)

I am proposing here that the role of language in communication first evolved as a side effect of its basic role in the construction of reality. The fact that communication is so central to our present view of language does not affect the argument. It is, in fact, theoretically elegant to explain the evolution of an important novel adaptation in a species by relating it to the conservation of earlier patterns of adaptation. We can think of language as being merely an expression of another neural contribution to the construction of mental imagery, analogous to the contributions of the encephalized sensory systems and their association systems. We need language more to tell stories than to direct actions. In the telling we create mental images in our listeners that might normally be produced only by the memory of events as recorded and integrated by the sensory and perceptual systems of the brain.

Mental images should be as real, in a fundamental sense, as the immediately experienced real world. Both are constructions of the brain, although it is appropriate to encode them in order to distinguish image from reality. The role of language in human communication is special because we have the vocal and manual apparatus to create spoken and written language. In hearing or reading another's words we literally share another's consciousness, and it is that familiar use of language that is unique to man. The point, however, is that it was necessary to have a brain that created the kind of consciousness communicated by the motor mechanisms of language. That new capacity required an enormous amount of neural tissue, and much of the expansion of the human brain resulted from the development of language and related capacities for mental imagery.

The vertebrate brain evolved to control the normal range of behavior within each vertebrate species. It is reasonable to identify the brain of lower vertebrates as being adapted to control fixed-action patterns in response to specific patterns of stimulation, with few requirements for plasticity or flexibility. In the higher vertebrates, the birds and the mammals, plasticity and flexibility are evident in all living species. Yet the birds developed in their own direction, perfecting the fixed-action pattern as the basic behavioral response to environmental requirements. It is among the mammals that more flexible patterns of behavior have been the rule. If one defines intelligence as the capacity to construct perceptual worlds in which sensory information from various modalities is integrated as information about objects in space and time, the evolution of intelligence is most evident in mammals. That capacity was most elaborately developed in the primates, a group of mammals adapted toward adaptability. In the primates skeletal specialization was minimal and adaptations were more completely determined by the enlargement of the brain and the development of learned-behavior mechanisms than they were in any other vertebrates. The trend culminated in man, and we know it as the capacity for imagery, for language and for culture.

The Organization of the Brain

The brain and spinal cord of mammals, including man, consist of some billions of neurons, and a single neuron may connect with thousands of others. How is this enormous three-dimensional network organized?

. . .

Walle J. H. Nauta and Michael Feirtag
September, 1979

We see two broadside approaches to the presentation of neuroanatomy. The first one is heroic: it affirms that the brain is the embodient of thinking and feeling and wanting, of learning and memory and of that curious sense that human beings share, a sense of the future. Then one contemplates this mystery made flesh. Certain parts of the brain, most notably the cerebral cortex, are wonderfully organized; others are startling in their seeming disarray (see Figure 2.1). Yet even the most highly ordered structures, with neurons and their various interconnections aligned as if on circuit boards, resist our present understanding.

The other approach is more matter-of-fact. The brain plainly has divisions, because the appropriate staining techniques reveal aggregations of neurons embedded in a feltwork of their filamentous extensions (see Figure 2.2). Moreover, in other places the tissue is composed primarily of the long nerve-cell fibers—the axons—that subserve long-distance communications in the nervous system. The first kind of tissue is gray matter, the second is white matter.

One is of course tempted to assign a function to each district, as if the entire brain were something like a radio. Yet the essence of the central nervous system—the brain and the spinal cord—is a channeling of incoming sensory information to a multiplicity of structures and a convergence of information on the neurons that animate the effector tissues of the body: the muscles and the glands. The overall system therefore assumes properties beyond those to be discovered in a mere set of modules.

Consider the brain structure named the subthalamic nucleus. Its destruction in the human brain leads to the motor dysfunction known as hemiballism, in which the patient uncontrollably makes motions that resemble the throwing of a ball. Is the normal function of the intact subthalamic nucleus therefore the suppression of motions resembling the throwing of a ball? Of course not; the condition represents only the action of a central nervous system unbalanced by the absence of a subthalamic nucleus.

We mention these things to establish the limitations of any account of the anatomy of the brain. We shall give such an account here, but it will necessarily be somewhat shadowy. To suggest otherwise would simply not be frank.

Some preliminaries will be useful. In the early decades of this century George Parker of Yale University had been searching for the primeval reflex arc. Such arcs had been identified in vertebrate animals; they are pathways consisting of one or more neurons by which the excitatory event elicited by a sensory stimulus to some part of the body can be conducted to an effector tissue and thereby can entail a movement. In Parker's time reflex arcs were commonly taken to be the simplest pattern by which nature had organized cells into a nervous system; accordingly the nervous system was widely supposed to have originated when some organism came to have a cell, or chain of cells, that mediated between an environmental stimulus and the organism's responsive movement. Presumably it would one day be established that the evolution of the nervous system had brought forth, in ever more advanced organisms, an ever increasing number and complexity of such chains.

Parker's attention was drawn first to the epithelial layer of certain marine polyps and sea anemones, because it contained an occasional cell that stood out (when it was appropriately stained) as if it were a neuron. At the base of such a cell Parker could see the beginning of a filament, looking rather like an axon, that broke up into end branches as it approached a muscle fiber. He could not be certain that the two made contact, but he assumed that there was communication between them. Surely he was right, but the arrangement is quite primitive; its circuitry could be called a one-neuron nervous system, since the entire line of conduction consists of only a single cell. What such a nervous system will do in response to a stimulus is as predictable as what a doorbell will do when the button is pressed. What is plain about the human nervous system, however, is that the behavior it makes human beings capable of is least of all predictable.

Obviously something must intervene in the doorbell mechanism, and so Parker examined the situation in somewhat more complex organisms. In certain polyps and jellyfishes he found an array of neurons in the epithelial layer similar to the array he had found earlier. Under the epithelium, however, he now found additional neurons that together form a widely distributed plexus. The nervous system in this second group of organisms has thereby gained in sophistication: neurons in the epithelial layer make contact with a subepithelial net, and the cells of that net make contact in turn with contractile tissue in the depths of the organism. One may

Figure 2.1 ORDER AND DISORDER in the cellular organization of the brain are apparent in these micrographs of thin sections of cat brain that were stained with two procedures: the Golgi stain, which causes only about 5 percent of the neurons to stand out in black silhouette, and the Nissl stain, which renders every neuronal cell body blue. (Here the blue is purplish.) The top micrograph shows the dentate gyrus of the hippocampus. Each neuronal cell body is an elongated pyramid aligned with its neighbors and extending its fibers in a parallel array. The bottom micrograph is of the magnocellular reticular formation. Here neurons are organized as an irregular net. Magnification of micrographs is 43 diameters. (Micrographs by Fritz Goro.)

therefore speak of a two-neuron nervous system, in which sensory neurons (in these simple creatures the neurons at the body surface, in direct contact with the organism's ambient environment) communicate with motor neurons (neurons that make contact with effector cells, in this instance contractile cells and therefore in essence muscle fibers).

Is this not circuitry that remains extremely predictable? Perhaps not. Imagine that the motor neurons communicate with one another, so that the input to any one of them includes not only messages coming from the ambient environment by way of sensory neurons but also messages from neighboring motor neurons. Imagine further that some messages might be excitatory, making the motor neuron more likely to generate and transmit its own activity if other signals should arrive, and that other messages might be inhibitory. Under such circumstances there is a riddle to solve: predicting what a neuron will do in response to its various inputs seems to be a matter of algebraically summing the excitatory and inhibitory messages that converge on it.

Perhaps the two-neuron arrangement enables the jellyfish so favored by nature to be more unpredictable in its behavior than the anemone and other organisms with one-neuron nervous systems. Then, however, comes a further advance, and it too is found in very primitive organisms, such as certain other jellyfishes. In a way it is the final advance, because the nervous system of these latter jellyfishes and the nervous system of man both consist in essence of only three classes of neurons. In these jellyfishes, as in man, the sensory neurons as a rule no longer communicate directly with motor neurons. Between the two has developed a barrier of neurons that have interconnections not only with motor neurons but also with one another.

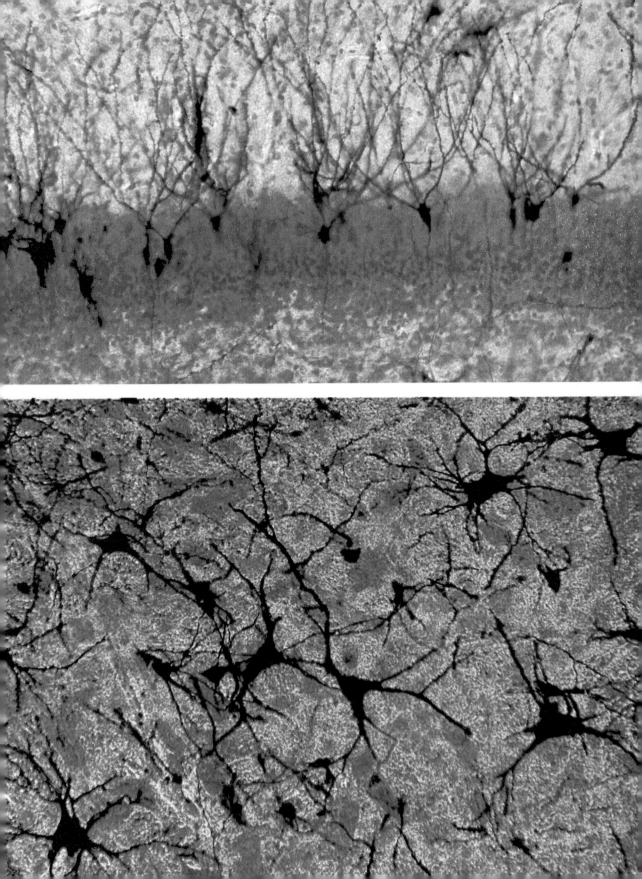

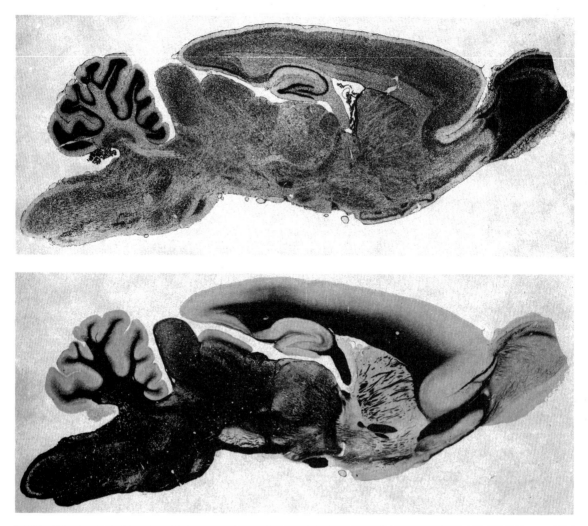

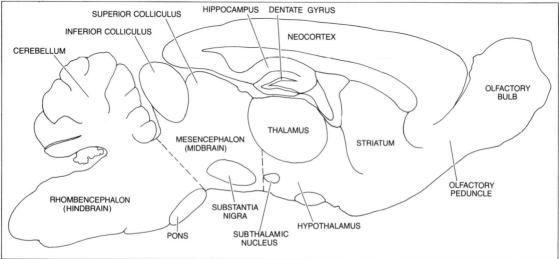

CEREBELLUM

INFERIOR COLLICULUS

SUPERIOR COLLICULUS

HIPPOCAMPUS DENTATE GYRUS

NEOCORTEX

OLFACTORY BULB

MESENCEPHALON (MIDBRAIN)

THALAMUS

STRIATUM

RHOMBENCEPHALON (HINDBRAIN)

SUBSTANTIA NIGRA

HYPOTHALAMUS

OLFACTORY PEDUNCLE

PONS

SUBTHALAMIC NUCLEUS

Figure 2.2 TWO STAINING TECHNIQUES provide complementary views of the internal organization of the rat brain. The section at the top, made just off the midplane and parallel to it, was treated by the Nissl technique, which selectively stains cell bodies. Each dot in the micrograph therefore corresponds to an individual cell. The section in the middle was treated with the Loyez technique, which selectively stains myelinated fibers and leaves cell bodies unstained, selectively revealing the fiber pathways. Map indicates the various anatomical structures. (Micrographs by Henry F. Hall and Diane Major.)

To be sure, this third and final step may already have been taken by all organisms that have a subepithelial nerve-cell plexus. In the foregoing account of a two-neuron nervous system all the cells composing that plexus were assumed to be motor neurons: cells that innervate effector tissues. In reality, however, only some of the many subepithelial cells may make such connections. The remainder may be positioned in the plexus in such a way that they receive input from the sensory neurons in the epithelium but can communicate only with others of their kind or with motor neurons, not with effector tissue. Neither sensory nor motoric, they are go-betweens in the path of sensory-to-motor conduction.

In short, here too are "intermediate neurons." Although a three-neuron organization is difficult to identify in a diffuse neuronal net, it is abundantly apparent at later stages in evolution; in animals more highly developed than a jellyfish the diffuse subepithelial nerve-cell plexus has been concentrated into either a segmental sequence of ganglia (aggregates of neurons) or a single unsegmented central nervous system. The crucial point is therefore the advent of "the great intermediate net": a barrier of intermediate neurons that interposes itself between the sensory neurons and the motor neurons early in the evolution of animal life.

Just how far the development of the great intermediate net has progressed to this day is best shown by some numbers. To begin with, how many neurons are there in the human central nervous system? One often hears that the answer is on the order of 10^{10}. This is an accounting of the intermediate and motor neurons, since it happens that the true sensory neurons lie not in the central nervous system but in ganglia that flank the brain and the spinal cord. It is an attractive number, easy to remember and easy to state. Yet there are classes of neurons so small and so densely crowded that it is

difficult or impossible to judge their number. One such class is the granule cell. There are so many granule cells in just one part of the human brain — the cerebellum — that the estimate of 10^{10} neurons in the entire central nervous system becomes suspect. The total could easily be an order of magnitude, perhaps two orders of magnitude, higher.

Still, assume for a moment that the total is 10^{10} How many of these cells are motor neurons? It appears that the answer cannot be many more than two or three million, which is a disconcertingly small number in view of the fact that only through motor neurons can the workings of the nervous system find expression in movement. Moreover, this answer suggests that an incredibly large number of influences must converge on the motor neurons; it suggests, in other words, that a typical motor neuron forms synapses with an enormous number of axons put out by an equally enormous number of neurons in the great intermediate net.

It is thought that a typical motor neuron in the human spinal cord has perhaps 10,000 synaptic contacts on its surface, of which about 2,000 are on the cell body and 8,000 are on its dendrites: its local branchings, as distinct from its single axon. This does not mean that 10,000 intermediate neurons impinge on one motor neuron; the intermediate neurons tend to make multiple synaptic contacts when they communicate with a cell. Even so, the average motor neuron must be heavily impinged on; a neuron count of 10^{10} in the central nervous system implies that for every motor neuron there are between 3,000 and 5,000 neurons of the great intermediate net.

One last conclusion must be drawn from the numbers we have quoted: the entire human brain and spinal cord are a great intermediate net, with the exception of a mere few million motor neurons. And when the great intermediate net comes to include 99.98 percent of all the neurons that make up the central nervous system, the term loses much of its meaning: it comes to represent the very complexity one must face in trying to comprehend the nervous system. The term remains useful only as a reminder that most of the brain's neurons are neither sensory nor motor. Strictly speaking, they are intercalated between the true sensory side of the organization and the true motoric side. They are the components of a computational network.

A second set of preliminaries concerns the gross anatomy of the central nervous system. In particular

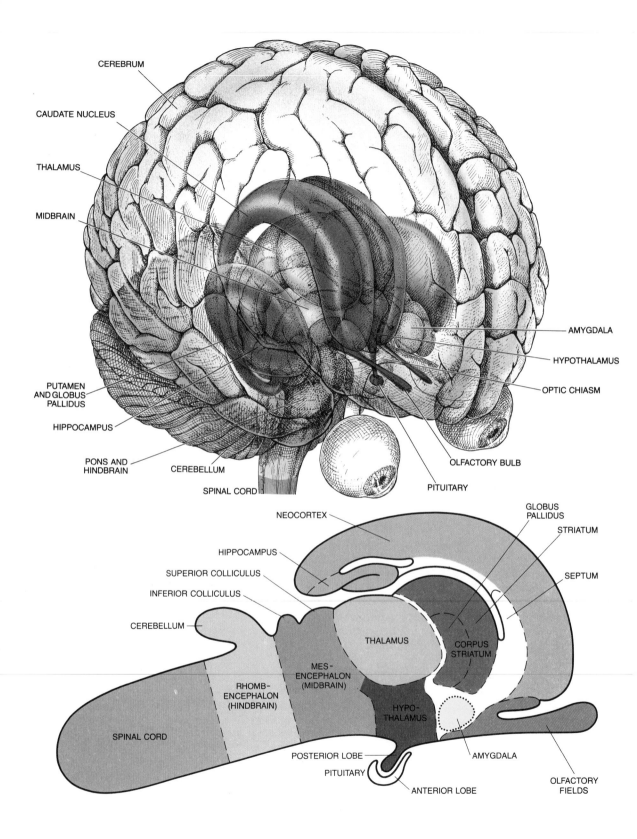

CEREBRUM

CAUDATE NUCLEUS

THALAMUS

MIDBRAIN

PUTAMEN
AND GLOBUS
PALLIDUS

HIPPOCAMPUS

PONS AND
HINDBRAIN

CEREBELLUM

SPINAL CORD

AMYGDALA

HYPOTHALAMUS

OPTIC CHIASM

OLFACTORY BULB

PITUITARY

NEOCORTEX

HIPPOCAMPUS

SUPERIOR COLLICULUS

INFERIOR COLLICULUS

CEREBELLUM

GLOBUS
PALLIDUS

STRIATUM

SEPTUM

RHOMB-
ENCEPHALON
(HINDBRAIN)

MES-
ENCEPHALON
(MIDBRAIN)

THALAMUS

CORPUS
STRIATUM

HYPO-
THALAMUS

SPINAL CORD

POSTERIOR LOBE

PITUITARY

ANTERIOR LOBE

AMYGDALA

OLFACTORY
FIELDS

Figure 2.3 A HUMAN BRAIN has been drawn so that its internal structures are visible through "transparent" outer layers of the cerebrum. At the bottom a generalized mammalian brain is shown in a highly schematic view. Corresponding structures in the realistic and schematic models are the same color. The hindbrain includes the cerebellum. The midbrain includes the two elevations known as the inferior and superior colliculi. The outer part of the forebrain is the cerebral hemisphere, the surface of which is the convoluted sheet of the cerebral cortex, which incorporates the hippocampus, the neocortex and the olfactory fields. Within the hemisphere are the amygdala and corpus striatum; the latter includes the globus pallidus and the striatum, which includes the caudate nucleus and putamen. The rest of the forebrain is the diencephalon: the upper two-thirds comprises the thalamus (which has numerous subdivisions) and the lower third the hypothalamus (which connects to pituitary complex).

the brain and spinal cord of all vertebrate species first appear in the embryo as no more than a tube only one cell layer thick. The anterior part of this neural tube, ultimately to be enclosed within the cranium, soon shows a series of three swellings: the primary brain vesicles. These are the rhombencephalon, or hindbrain; the mesencephalon, or midbrain, and the prosencephalon, or forebrain. (The suffix -encephalon is from the Greek for "within the head.")

Of the three primary vesicles the prosencephalon is the most productive in terms of both further subdivision and further differentiation. The major event in its embryonic development is the formation of chambers on its left and right sides. These become the paired cerebral hemispheres, also called the telencephalon or endbrain, which in some species are of modest size but in others are enormous. Between the hemispheres lies the unpaired central component of the prosencephalon from which the hemispheres diverge. It is called the diencephalon, which literally means "between-brain."

Concurrent with these developments the prosencephalon grows a further pair of chambers: the optic vesicles. Even sightless animals have them, but in animals that can see they elongate toward the surface of the head and ultimately become the two retinas, connected to the base of the forebrain by their stalks, the optic nerves. Lastly the underside of the primary prosencephalon develops an unpaired midline chamber that differentiates to form the posterior lobe of the pituitary complex.

Figure 2.3 suggests the outcome of these embryonic unfoldings. At the bottom of the figure is a schematic diagram that by and large holds for all mammals, and it depicts the fully formed mammalian central nervous system broken down into several subdivisions. At the left is the spinal cord greatly foreshortened in the figure. To its right, without any abrupt transition, is the rhombencephalon, the lowermost division of the brain itself. Its dorsal part (the part nearest the back of the animal) is the appendage called the cerebellum.

Above the rhombencephalon is the mesencephalon, which in mammals includes two pairs of structures that together form a region of four hills known as the lamina quadrigemina, the tectum mesencephali or simply the tectum, meaning roof. The lower pair of structures are the inferior colliculi. The upper pair are the superior colliculi. Other than that the mesencephalon gives little reason to subdivide it, at least in the longitudinal direction. It is in fact a rather short stretch of the human brain.

Next is the central, unpaired division of the forebrain, namely the diencephalon. Its dorsal two-thirds is the thalamus. The rest is the hypothalamus. (Somewhat off to the side of the hypothalamus is a third district of the diencephalon, the subthalamus, whose most striking cell group, the subthalamic nucleus, we mentioned at the beginning. Its inclusion here would overcrowd the figure.) The hypothalamus is characterized by the glandular appendage called the pituitary complex. It is also continuous in the forward direction with the septum, a structure that is best classified, in spite of its position, as being diencephalic.

The remaining subdivision of the forebrain is the telencephalon, the cerebral hemisphere. In the brain of a mammal it is by far the largest part, and in many mammalian species its shell, the cerebral mantle or cerebral cortex, is furrowed into the convolutions called gyri and the fissures called sulci. The mammalian cerebral cortex can be subdivided into several districts. At the base of the hemisphere a structure protrudes forward that is composed entirely of cortex, although it is cortex of a primitive cell architecture. Its swollen front end is the olfactory bulb and its shank is the olfactory peduncle; only the part immediately under the rest of the cerebral hemisphere is the olfactory cortex proper. A second great district of the mammalian cerebral cortex is found at the free edge of the cortex, where the cortical mantle rolls inward on itself to form a

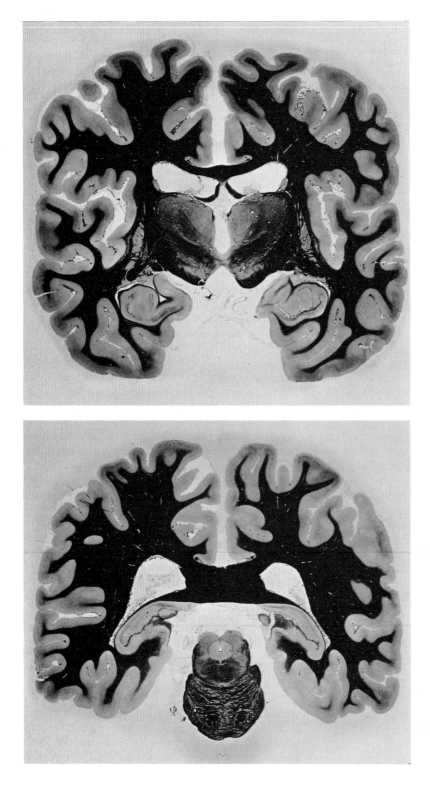

2.4 TWO SLICES through a fixed human brain perpendicular to its long axis. The staining selectively blackens the fatty myelin sheath of the nerve fibers; the white matter appears black and the gray matter is more or less unstained. The empty spaces indicate the location of the ventricles: fluid-filled cisterns deep within the brain. The top slice was made near the middle of the length of the brain and includes the cerebral cortex, the hippocampus and the thalamus. The bottom slice was made more to the rear and includes a section through the brain stem. Specimens are from the collection of Professor Paul I. Yakovlev at the Harvard Medical School. (See also Figure 2.5.)

composite gyrus whose cross section is reminiscent of a rococo ornament. This remarkable structure is known as the hippocampus. (See Figures 2.3, 2.4 and 2.5.)

There remains even after the foregoing parcellation an expanse of the mammalian cerebral cortex that has enormous extent and structural complexity; in man and other primates it is estimated to contain no fewer than 70 percent of all the neurons in the central nervous system. This is the neocortex. It is the latest form of cortex to appear in evolution. We owe it to a branching; beyond the reptiles one strain of animals elaborated on the reptilian pattern and became the birds, while a more venturesome strain developed the neocortex as it became the mammals. From a strictly phylogenetic point of view birds are thus the logical end of the brain's traditional development and the mammals are deviants, since there

are no birds in their ancestry. In one of the many radiations of mammalian evolution the primates appeared, an order in which the neocortex reaches its maximal development. We human beings are heir to all the consequences, perhaps including psychiatry.

In the depths of the mammalian cerebral hemisphere are several masses of gray matter. One is the amygdala, which lies under the olfactory cortex. Another is the corpus striatum, at the very core of the cerebral hemisphere. It consists in turn of two districts that are distinct in cell composition. The first of these is an inner zone called the pallidum or globus pallidus. The other is an outer district known as the striatum.

We turn now to the circuitry of the mammalian central nervous system. Let us begin with an identification of sensory neurons, such as those

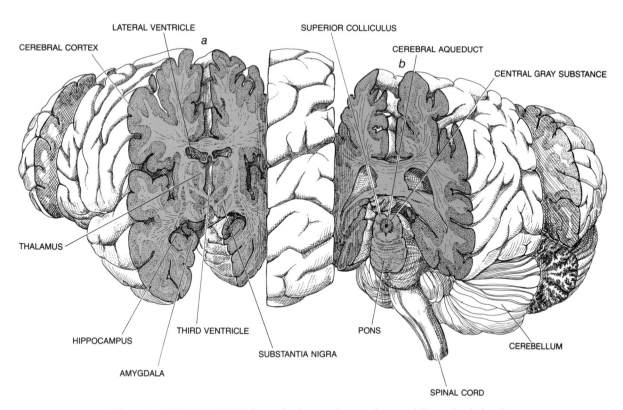

Figure 2.5 HUMAN BRAIN is cut in five sections and opened like a book for the purpose of correlating its external and internal anatomy. The two slices in Figure 2.4 are designated *a* and *b*. At the level of slice *b* the brain stem lies below the mass of the forebrain.

Parker found in the epithelial layer of jellyfishes. In vertebrates, however, the position of the sensory neurons is quite different. Only one known instance remains in which a vertebrate's sensory neuron is also a receptor at the surface of the body; only the olfactory epithelial cells, in the lining of the roof of the nasal cavity, are exposed to the external environment. All other sensory neurons in the body of a vertebrate are stationed well below the surface, in ganglia along the length of the spinal cord or in similar ganglia flanking the brain. (In vertebrates the term ganglion is reserved for a cluster of neurons outside the central nervous system.) Each sensory neuron has an axon that divides into two parts: one part enters the central nervous system and the other innervates structures of the periphery.

In Figure 2.6 one of these cells—let us call it a primary sensory neuron—sends an axon into the spinal cord bearing reports of somatic sensory events such as a touch on the skin, the movment of a joint or the contraction of a muscle. These messages do not immediately reach motor neurons; the primary sensory neuron makes its first synaptic contacts with what are called intermediate neurons.

There is, however, an exception. It is the monosynaptic reflex arc, in which a side branch from a primary sensory fiber bridges over and makes direct synaptic contact on a motor neuron. At first this seems dismaying: only a few paragraphs above we noted that after the earliest stages of neural evolution motor neurons no longer were bothered with raw data. We suggested they were instead always given digests of information by neurons of the great intermediate net. A monosynaptic reflex might therefore seem to be a very primitive type of neural circuitry. On the other hand, it could be fairly new; perhaps only terrestrial animals have redeveloped it. Air and land, after all, are the cruelest of environments; for a mountain goat one misstep could be fatal. A fish, in contrast, can make any number of similar faux pas and not be harmed in any way. The fish is splendidly suspended; the force of gravity is not nearly so stringent and hostile. Hence it is terrestrial life, not aquatic, that seems to require a high-security reflex system for maintaining balance, and specifically a way in which a muscle can signal to the appropriate motor neurons (and only the appropriate ones) that it is being unduly stretched by the force of gravity.

Monosynaptic reflex arcs have never been found outside the realm of such corrections. Thus the short circuits between sensory input and motor output

appear to be a small minority. The large majority of mammalian primary sensory fibers enter the great intermediate net and synapse with members of what we shall call a secondary sensory cell group: neurons first in line to receive primary sensory input. From there many pathways are directed more or less promptly toward motor neurons. They might collectively be called a local reflex channel, if it is kept in mind that "local" may be misleading because there are several reflexes that involve the entire length of the spinal cord but nonetheless are local because they remain within it. The first link in the local reflex channel is a cell of the secondary sensory cell group. Many such cells do not themselves make contact with a motor neuron; they synapse instead on yet other neurons of the great intermediate net, and it is only these latter neurons that finally complete the arc.

Other channels consist of axons not directed toward motor neurons. Take the cerebellar channel: from secondary sensory cell groups in the hindbrain and spinal cord there are many axons ascending directly to the cerebellum. The axon that does so in Figure 2.6 originates in a secondary sensory cell group of the spinal cord and is therefore called a spino-cerebellar fiber. ("Axon" and "fiber" are synonymous in neuroanatomical usage.) Many of these fibers together would compose a spinocerebellar tract or bundle.

A third channel is the lemniscal channel. The word lemniscus is Latin for ribbon, and it refers here to fiber bundles that originate in secondary sensory cell groups and ascend toward the forebrain, in particular toward the thalamus. In Figure 2.6 one such bundle is shown ascending at the center of the spinal cord. Actually it ascends near the cord's lateral edge; the simple scheme of Figure 2.6 cannot be topographic. The bundle is called the spinothalamic tract, although only one of its three representative fibers is depicted as arriving at the thalamus. The other fibers accompany it for some distance and then crash-land, so to speak: both are shown terminating on neurons in the rhombencephalon, although one or the other might just as well have terminated somewhat farther forward, in the mesencephalon. The point is that of the spinothalamic fibers only a small fraction actually reach the thalamus. Even so the tract is named after the successful minority, which terminate in a specific part of the thalamus: the ventral nucleus. Here the fibers synapse with thalamic neurons whose axons travel

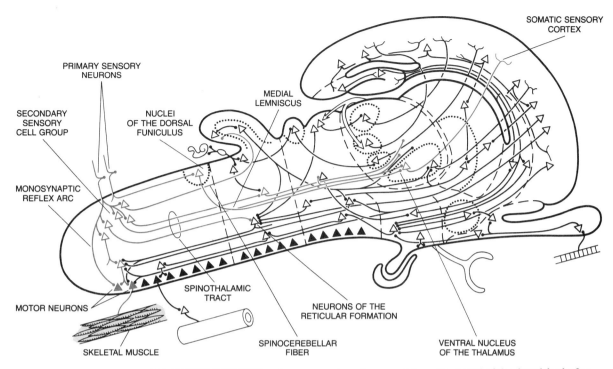

Figure 2.6 SOMATIC SENSORY INFORMATION such as skin sensation is transmitted along several spinal pathways. At the left a representative pair of primary sensory neurons deliver signals from peripheral sensory receptors into the spinal cord (SC). One path branches immediately to motor neurons (*solid triangles*), whose fibers lead outward to the skeletal musculature. All the other paths lead initially to secondary sensory cell groups, in the SC or nuclei of the dorsal funiculus. The medial lemniscus pathway travels upward from the nuclei of the dorsal funiculus to the ventral nucleus of the thalamus, which in turn projects to the somatic sensory area of the cortex. The spinothalamic tract travels upward to the forebrain from the secondary cell groups throughout the length of the spinal cord, sending out fibers en route. A small fraction of the spinothalamic-tract fibers ultimately reach the ventral nucleus. The secondary cell groups also send fibers to the cerebellum.

without interruption to a specific field of neocortex, a field that is known as the somatic sensory cortex.

Note that the path from a primary sensory neuron to the neocortex in this case involves only two synaptic interruptions. The first is in the spinal cord, between a primary sensory fiber and a neuron in a secondary sensory cell group. The second interruption is in the diencephalon, between a lemniscal fiber and a neuron in the ventral nucleus of the thalamus. What happens in the neocortex, however, is a synaptic cataclysm. In the neocortex the response to an arriving signal initially involves hundreds or even thousands of neurons. And acting through synaptic connections, the first neurons engaged by the signal will engage innumerable further neurons.

A two-synapse sensory conduction line to the neocortex might be called a through line, because two synapses appears to be a minimum in such systems. It might also be called a closed or labeled line, because in general the sensory pathways of minimal interruption rigorously maintain the topography of the sensory periphery from which they come. A fingertip, for example, can detect two distinct stimuli when it is touched by the points of a pair of drafting dividers no more than two or three millimeters apart. This ability is called two-point discrimination. Its existence means that each of the compass points must stimulate paths of conduction that are independent enough to allow what might be called sensory resolution. Some cell in the somatic sensory cortex, if interrogated with a microelectrode, might reveal that its only interest is a square millimeter of skin on the index finger. One of its close neighbors might be the monitor of an adjoining square millimeter, and so on. In that way the topography of the body surface would be faithfully reproduced.

A conduction path diametrically opposed to one that is "labeled" would be one in which the line becomes involved in the conduction of topographically muddled messages from a given sensorium, or even messages from several different sensoria. This curious arrangement in fact exists: one of the spinothalamic dropouts in Figure 2.6 ends in synaptic contact with a rhombencephalic neuron whose axon continues the line into the thalamus. At that extra interruption, however, the line accepts messages not only from the spinothalamic fiber but also from the auditory system.

How can the thalamus know what has happened when an impulse arrives by way of this system? The rhombencephalic neuron is called multimodal or nonspecific, and the conduction path might be called open-line: wherever there is a synaptic interruption the line is open to inputs from other neurons. The great majority of neurons in the core of the hindbrain and midbrain are of this curious nonspecific nature. They sit with their dendrites— their cellular hands—spread across several millimeters, hoping, it seems, to catch any kind of message. They are typical of what is called the reticular formation, where relatively few cell groups receive homogeneous inputs.

An electrical engineer who had this situation described to him might frown; he would say that one could never hope to get anything but noise from it. The situation nonetheless prevails in the brains of all vertebrates, including man. Its existence would therefore seem to correspond to some particular need. At the moment it seems permissible to say that the reticular formation includes among its functions the production of a background of general arousal in the central nervous system and that the formation embodies a mechanism by which activity states throughout the central nervous system are regulated. Some of these regulations are diurnal; one state is sleep, another is wakefulness. Between the two there are a great many shadings of alertness and inattentiveness. All are expressions of one or another pattern of activity in the reticular formation.

Surely the electrical engineer would more happily contemplate a second somatic sensory lemniscus

rising from the spinal cord. This is the medial lemniscus. It is far more tightly organized: almost all its fibers are labeled lines that ascend directly to the ventral nucleus of the thalamus from a pair of secondary sensory cell groups at the transition between the spinal cord and the hindbrain that are called the nuclei of the dorsal funiculus. The engineer would not be surprised to learn that two-point discrimination is represented far more prominently in the medial lemniscus than it is in the spinothalamic tract.

What of the other sensoria? The little organ that appears for diagrammatic convenience near the cerebellum in Figure 2.7 is the organ of hearing. Within it cells that have a single cilium are found in a highly specialized epithelial complex called Corti's organ. They are innervated by primary sensory neurons whose centrally directed processes terminate on neurons of the cochlear nuclei, a secondary sensory cell group in the rhombencephalon specializing in the reception and processing of afflux exclusively from the auditory sensorium. Figure 2.7 shows only two such neurons; actually there are tens of thousands. From the cochlear nuclei originates the lateral lemniscus, ascending toward the thalamus. None of its fibers extend beyond the inferior colliculus. In this unbypassable way station in the mesencephalon axons originate that do attain the thalamus, where they terminate in the medial geniculate body. (Not shown in Figure 2.7 are several other auditory way stations, apparently more optional, associated with the lateral lemniscus itself.) The neurons of the medial geniculate body in turn project—send their axons—to the specific area of the neocortex called the auditory cortex.

Compare this with the visual system. A multitude of neurons in the retina process the output of the eye's photoreceptor apparatus. The axons of certain of these cells first form the optic nerve. Then comes a rechanneling of axons in which those entrained by the nasal half of each retina cross the midplane of the head to join those entrained by the lateral half of the other eye's retina. The result is the optic tract. Each optic tract distributes its constituent axons to two great terminal areas. One is the superior colliculus, but in all primates the more important area, at least in terms of the number of axons, is the lateral geniculate body of the thalamus. The neurons of that group of cells project in turn to the neocortex, specifically to an area at the posterior pole of the cerebral hemisphere that is known as the visual cortex.

Note that whereas no auditory fiber can reach its thalamic way station without synaptic interruption, most visual fibers (in primates) can. It should be added, however, that many of the neurons in the superior colliculus that receive visual fibers send their own axons into the thalamus, not to the lateral geniculate body but to the nucleus lateralis posterior. The neurons of this latter cell group in turn project to the neocortex. They project, however, not to the area in which axons entrained by the lateral geniculate body terminate but to a nearby cortical region that is distinct from the visual cortex. The visual system apparently has two channels ascending to the cerebral cortex.

The olfactory system breaks all the laws that seem to govern the organization of other sensory mechanisms. It is, as we have noted, the only system known in which the primary sensory neurons lie at the body surface. There is no transducing element, as there is in, say, Corti's organ; the olfactory epithelial cell itself is buffeted by the external environment. From such a neuron a very thin axon projects to the olfactory bulb, whose neurons in turn give rise to axons that terminate in synaptic contact on cells in the olfactory cortex.

We now have traced the fibers of four sensoria: the somatic sensorium and the sensoria of hearing, vision and olfaction. A number of conclusions may by now have begun to emerge. For one thing, the thalamus appears to be a crucial way station, a final checkpoint, before messages from all the sensoria (except, it seems, olfaction) are allowed entrance to

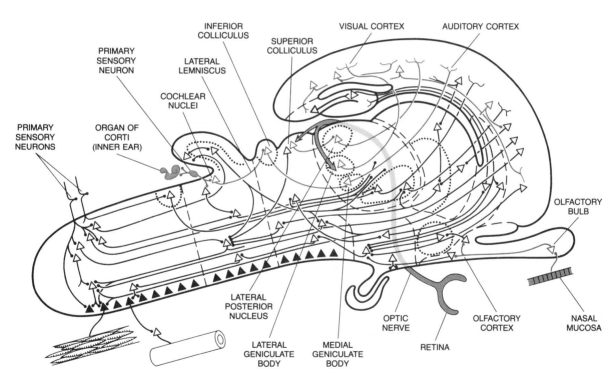

Figure 2.7 THREE SENSORIA (hearing, vision and olfaction) send their information to the cerebral cortex in different ways. The pathways for hearing pass successively through the cochlear nuclei of the hindbrain, the inferior colliculus of the midbrain and the medial geniculate body of the thalamus before they reach the auditory area of the cerebral cortex. The pathways for vision begin in the retina (which is actually a part of the brain) and then enter two different channels: one traveling by way of the lateral geniculate body in the thalamus to the visual cortex, the other projecting by way of the superior colliculus in the midbrain to a way station in the thalamus and then to a cortical area near the visual cortex. In the olfactory system the receptor neurons in the nasal mucosa project without the mediation of the thalamus to the olfactory bulb, which is a part of the cerebral cortex. The olfactory bulb then projects in turn to the olfactory cortex proper.

higher stations of the brain. It is tempting to call any such interruption a relay, but what happens at these breaks in neural circuitry can be far more than what happens in an athletic relay where each runner hands a baton to the next and the baton arrives unmodified at the end of the course. In the central nervous system the "relay" is entirely different. At each synaptic interruption in a sensory pathway the input is transformed: the code in which the message arrived is fundamentally changed. Presumably the data could not be understood at higher levels; translation is needed, and the synaptic relays are better spoken of as processing stations.

Then there is the conclusion that the cerebral cortex is an end station of the sensory conduction pathways. The neuroanatomist is highly satisfied when he can trace the visual system, for example, from the retina to the lateral geniculate body and from there to the visual cortex. The problem with any further tracing is the complexity of the cerebral cortex, with its 70 percent of all the neurons in the human central nervous system. What are they doing with their input? Two observations might be offered.

First, the thalamocortical projections are reciprocated: the visual cortex projects back to the lateral geniculate body, from which it received its input; the auditory cortex projects back to the medial geniculate body, and the somatic sensory cortex projects back to the medial geniculate body, and the somatic sensory cortex projects back to the ventral nucleus. This reciprocity undoubtedly signifies that the functional state of the cortex can influence the manner in which the sensory way stations of the thalamus screen the cortically directed flow of information.

Second, the visual, auditory and somatic sensory areas embody only a first cortical step in the sensory processing. Out from these primary sensory fields come fibers that synaptically affect adjoining areas that cannot unreservedly be called sensory; they are a block away, so to speak, from the arriving input. And out from these areas come fibers that terminate in areas still farther away from the primary sensory fields. The areas of the neocortex at various removes from the primary fields are called association areas, and in man they represent by far the largest fraction of the cortical expanse: visual cortex, auditory cortex and somatic sensory cortex together account for only about a fourth of the total. More advanced stages of processing presumably are embodied in association cortex. For example, there are places

where the auditory and the visual converge. It is now known that the march of neural processing through the neocortex typically involves a sequence of association areas, and that a destination of the march seems invariably to be the hippocampus or the amygdala, or both.

In 1870 Gustav Theodor Fritsch and Eduard Hitzig published a report that electric current of minimal strength, applied to an area of the neocortex immediately in front of what is called the central sulcus, would elicit twitchings of skeletal (as opposed to visceral) musculature on the side of the body opposite the site of stimulation. Often it was the hand or foot that moved. This discovery, perhaps the first suggestion of a functional compartmentalization in the cerebral cortex, aroused an enduring interest in the organization of those parts of the brain involved in effector (or motor) functions. After all, here was a motor cortex: a circumscribed place at the highest level of the brain that plainly was implicated in bodily movement. Perhaps a purely motoric organization could now be dissected out, so to speak, throughout the brain and spinal cord.

So began the quest for the "motor system," a vague term designating not only the motor neurons governing the skeletal musculature but also the neural channels that converge on motor neurons. The quest continues to this day, and one may fairly ask whether it can ever be completed. Consider area 19, a band of neocortex distinct in cell architecture from neighboring zones and situated not far from the visual cortex. When area 19 is stimulated electrically in an experimental animal, the eyes of the animal turn in unison to the contralateral side, that is, the gaze moves to an alignment directed away from the side of the brain receiving the electric current. It is therefore tempting to call area 19 a "motor" area. To do so, however, would be arbitrary, because from another point of view area 19 is sensory: it is known to reprocess information that has passed through the visual cortex. A similar example is associated with the auditory sensorium: there is a locus designated area 22, near the auditory cortex proper, where electrical stimulation will again cause the animal to turn its eyes to the contralateral side. Yet area 22 stands in synaptic relation to the auditory cortex much as area 19 does to the visual cortex.

The lesson is that no line can be drawn between a sensory side and a motor side in the organization of the brain. To put it another way, all neural structures are involved in the programming and guidance of an organism's behavior. Surely that is in essence the function of the nervous system, and the reason evolution has favored its development. Of course, some structures lie within the great intermediate net in a way that encourages their identification as sensory; the lateral geniculate body of the thalamus is an example. To other structures, situated not too many synapses away from motor neurons, one is tempted to apply the label motor. That, however, is the only way in which either of these labels can reasonably be employed. Accordingly it may be best to explore the motor aspects of the central nervous system by beginning at the level of the motor neuron, which is unequivocally a part of the motor system by anyone's definition, and then attempting to trace into the brain the lines that play on it. Be aware, though, that following this strategy means moving upstream: against the prevailing direction of neural traffic.

The first step "upward" from the motor neuron is in general a short one, since the strongest force acting to guide a typical motor neuron seems to emanate from a pool of cells that usually are smaller and usually are nearby. Let us call the sum of all motor neurons and their guiding neuronal pools the "lower motor system," and let us divide this system into functional subunits, each called a "local motor apparatus," that correspond to the parts of the body: the arms, the legs, the eyes and so on. Each local motor apparatus is, it seems, a kind of file room in which blueprints, each one representing a possible movement of a particular body part, are stored. The brain, with its descending fiber systems, reaches down and selects the appropriate blueprint.

What, then, are the sources of the descending systems? What influences the local motor apparatus? Motor neurons lie within the spinal cord and the hindbrain and the midbrain; there are none in the forebrain. Here, however, we can consider only the projections that converge on the spinal cord. They originate at all levels of the central nervous system. Within the cord itself many of them originate in secondary sensory cell groups, or even, in the case of monosynaptic reflex arcs, as the collaterals of certain primary sensory fibers. Within the rhombencephalon the projections originate mainly in the inner two-thirds of the rhombencephalic reticular formation, a district known as the magnocellular reticular formation in recognition of its content

of large and very large neuronal cell bodies. Within the mesencephalon the projections originate in the superior colliculus and also in a large cell mass called the red nucleus. Generally speaking, all three of these fiber systems descending into the spinal cord (reticulospinal, tectospinal and rubrospinal tracts by name) must be seen as bearing information—commands, if you wish—that may have antecedents in wide regions of the brain. The superior colliculus receives input not only from the optic nerve but also from large areas of the cerebral cortex, including the visual cortex and much else. The red nucleus receives input primarily from the cerebellum and the motor cortex.

As for the reticular formation, it is particularly notable as a place of convergence for information of widespread origin. We suggested this above, of course, when we were speaking of ascending systems; it also applies here, in a context of descent. A neuron that represents it is shown in Figure 2.8; it is modeled on neurons whose electrical activity was recorded by Giuseppe Moruzzi at the University of Pisa and others. It lies in the rhombencephalic reticular formation, and it will respond, it seems, to inputs from a secondary sensory cell group in the spinal cord. A flash of light, however, may also provoke it, because a report of that event could conceivably reach the reticular formation by a descending path originating in the superior colliculus. Further still, the cell may respond to a message from the cerebellum, or from the neocortex, or from the mesencephalic reticular formation. In short, a large number of heterogeneous inputs converge on the cell. Clearly the reticular formation must integrate this vast variety of neural afflux, ascending and descending in the brain, and then it may dispatch impulses over reticulospinal fibers that terminate on spinal intermediate neurons, or even, although infrequently, on motor neurons directly. Perhaps the reader will hear again the outcry of the engineer that the reticular formation makes no engineering sense.

It now remains to superimpose on the encephalospinal systems of the hindbrain and midbrain the descending systems that have their origin in the forebrain. In the first place essentially all areas of the neocortex project to the striatum, the outer zone of the corpus striatum. The layout is a topographical one: the somatic sensory cortex projects to a striatal district distinct from that receiving the visual projection, or the auditory projection, or the projections

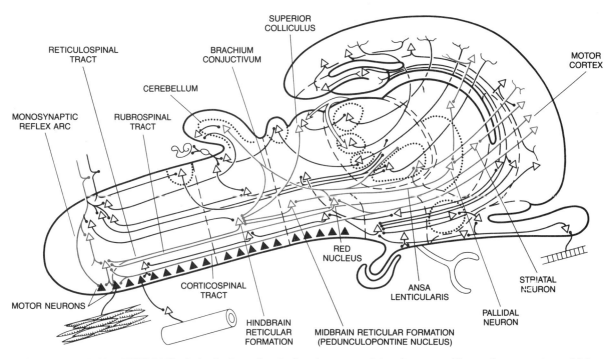

SUPERIOR COLLICULUS

RETICULOSPINAL TRACT

BRACHIUM CONJUCTIVUM

MOTOR CORTEX

CEREBELLUM

MONOSYNAPTIC REFLEX ARC

RUBROSPINAL TRACT

RED NUCLEUS

MOTOR NEURONS

CORTICOSPINAL TRACT

ANSA LENTICULARIS

STRIATAL NEURON

PALLIDAL NEURON

HINDBRAIN RETICULAR FORMATION

MIDBRAIN RETICULAR FORMATION (PEDUNCULOPONTINE NUCLEUS)

Figure 2.8 MOTOR NEURONS of the brain and spinal cord (*solid triangles*) receive information from highly convergent channels. Here motor neurons are shown receiving input from a primary sensory neuron, from a secondary sensory cell group in the spinal cord, from the reticular formation of the brain stem, from the red nucleus of the midbrain and from the motor cortex of the forebrain. The red nucleus and the reticular formation receive inputs from a variety of sources. The entire neocortex, which includes auditory, visual, somatic sensory and motor fields and other fields as well, sends projections to the corpus striatum. This cell mass projects its fibers in turn to the reticular formation, which ultimately acts on motor neurons. A second pathway from the corpus striatum serves as a feedback loop: it sends its fibers to a part of the thalamus that projects back again to the motor cortex.

from the association areas or from the motor cortex. From the striatum a massive projection converges on the globus pallidus (or pallidum), the inner division of the corpus striatum. There are many fewer neurons in the globus pallidus than there are in the striatum, so that this system must be seen as a kind of funneling.

From the globus pallidus the path continues downward in a fiber bundle called the ansa lenticularis, downward except for a curious exception: a large part of the ansa lenticularis curves back on itself and enters the upper part of the ventral nucleus. We have noted that this call mass of the thalamus receives the two great somatic sensory lemnisci, the medial lemniscus and the spinothalamic tract, and that it projects to the somatic sensory cortex. Only the posterior part of the ventral nucleus, however, is a somatic sensory way station.

The more forward part of the same cell group receives two large systems: the ansa lenticularis and the cerebellum's upward projection, the brachium conjunctivum. It too projects to neocortex, not to any sensory area but to the motor cortex.

Pathologies that disrupt this curious looping circuitry cause great havoc in bodily movements. One such pathology involves an input to the striatum that does not come from the cerebral cortex. It comes from a cell group in the midbrain whose neurons are pigmented; in man they are black even in unstained preparations. For that reason the cell group became known late in the 18th century as the substantia nigra, the black substance. Extensive loss of the black pigmented neurons causes the disorder of movement known as Parkinsonism. It is characterized by a muscular rigidity that greatly hampers movement and is betrayed by, among other things, a masklike face. There is also a peculiar tremor, of low frequency and almost rotatory, that affects the arms and hands. The patient's first complaint, however, is typically that he has difficulty initiating the movements he intends to make. He may want to adjust his clothing, but somehow he cannot start.

The corpus striatum can therefore be considered an important influence on bodily movement. To speak more broadly it can be regarded as one among the large number of brain structures whose output seems channeled toward motor neurons. Yet the remarkable fact remains that the corpus striatum cannot directly affect such neurons, or even directly affect the neuronal pools that act as their gatekeepers. We have just seen that a part of its outgoing tract, the ansa lenticularis, turns upward and enters the ventral nucleus of the thalamus. The rest of the ansa lenticularis continues downward past this turning but goes no farther than the caudal limit of the midbrain, where a single neuron in the illustration below symbolizes a group of several thousand neurons composing the pedunculopontine nucleus. It is a part of the mesencephalic reticular formation. From here the descending path becomes vague. The reticular formation is a site of formidable difficulty in both anatomical and functional analysis.

The projections from the neocortex to the striatum are by no means the only corticofugal fibers. As we have noted, some of the neocortical outflow terminates in the various thalamic nuclei and reciprocates the projections from the thalamus to the neocortex. Some penetrates into the midbrain, to terminate in the superior colliculus, the red nucleus and the mesencephalic reticular formation. Still another contingent, arising from all parts of the neocortex, makes its synapses in the pons, a district of the hindbrain, which projects in turn to the cerebellum. The remaining corticofugal fibers, the ones that extend beyond the pons, originate mostly in the motor cortex. Some of them will reach no farther than the rhombencephalic reticular formation; others will attain all levels of the spinal cord.

These latter fibers, which compose the corticospinal tract, are particularly noteworthy. It is remarkable in itself that they travel from the cortex to the spinal cord, since fibers descending from the corpus striatum get no farther than the midbrain. It also is remarkable that an estimated 5 percent of the corticospinal fibers synapse directly on motor neurons. That is a formidable bypass; these fibers

not only enter the spinal cord but also avoid the neuronal pools of the local motor apparatus. It turns out that they synapse preferentially on the motor neurons that animate the musculature of the extremities. Doubtless the existence of the corticospinal tract accounts for the observation that of all the areas of the cerebral cortex the motor cortex needs the least electrical stimulation to elicit experimental bodily movement. The explanation is that of all the areas of the cerebral cortex the motor cortex lies the fewest synapses away from motor neurons.

The motor system almost defies examination from the standpoint of volitional behavior, as opposed to nonvolitional. Consider a humiliating experience common among tennis players. The player makes a brilliant return and feels elated. Then he decides it was simply a fluke; the next time a tennis ball rushes at him with a similar trajectory he will probably hit it badly. It is true that a difficult volitional movement has been performed successfully, but does the person who performed it deserve any credit?

In spite of the enigma of volitional control, the subjective experience of volition has given a name to the motor system that innervates skeletal musculature: it is the voluntary, or somatic, nervous system, as distinguished from the involuntary, or autonomic, nervous system that innervates glands and the smooth musculature of the viscera. A misunderstanding is implicit in this latter nomenclature, however, just as surely as one was implicit in the former. It has to do with the term "autonomic," which means "self-governing." The autonomic nervous system is not self-governing at all. Its functions are integrated with voluntary movements no less than with motivations and affects. In short, its roots are in the brain: one's experiences from moment to moment dictate not only the contractions of one's skeletal muscles but also large functional shifts in the body's internal organs. The term autonomic has nonetheless won out in the English-speaking world. Other languages use other terms. In German one speaks of *das viszerale Nervensystem*, in French of *le système nerveux végétatif*.

The autonomic periphery is suggested in Figure 2.9 by a tubelike hollow organ, perhaps the intestinal tract or the urinary bladder or a bronchus or an artery; all are in essence tubelike structures whose width is determined by one or more coatings of smooth musculature. The motor innervation of such muscle tissue (or of gland) employs two neurons.

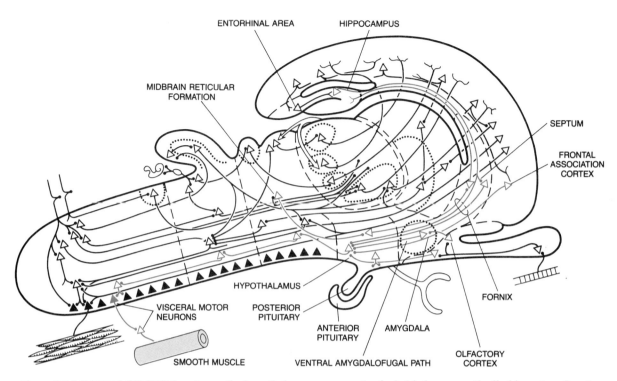

Figure 2.9 LOOPING CIRCUITS center on the hypothalamus, which regulates the activities of glands and smooth muscle (such as the involuntary muscle of the viscera) through the autonomic nervous system and the pituitary complex. The hypothalamus receives projections from the hippocampus and the amygdala, which are the principal components of what is known as the limbic system. Input to the hypothalamus also derives from the reticular formation. A further source of input is the frontal cortex, in the most forward part of the cerebral hemispheres. The limbic system is the destination for pathways from the cerebral cortex, including direct projections from olfactory cortex.

The first neuron lies within the central nervous system. It entrains a rather thin axon that synapses in the periphery on a second neuron, which is often situated in a ganglion. The second neuron in turn sends its axon to terminate in the visceral effector tissue.

Within the brain neurons that specifically affect the activity of the autonomic nervous system appear to be concentrated in the hypothalamus. The evidence is clear: When the hypothalamus of almost any animal, emphatically including man, is suddenly destroyed, its possessor dies, with upheavals in what Claude Bernard called the internal milieu, a term embracing tissue fluids and organ functions, as determined by blood pressure, heart rate, respiration rate and so on. Neurosurgeons obliged to operate near the hypothalamus therefore are always concerned lest the structure be so much as buffeted. Indeed, patients have died of hyperthermia (an acute rise in body temperature) after otherwise successful brain surgery in which caution about injuring the hypothalamus seems to have been exemplary. On the other hand, when a massive lesion of the hypothalamus develops slowly, perhaps in the form of a slow-growing tumor, there may be no dramatic effects at all. It is as if there were a chain of command in the autonomic nervous system, or, as Bernard put it, an automatism of levels: when the hypothalamus is slowly incapacitated, regions of the brain below the hypothalamus can keep the internal milieu stable, albeit within narrow limits.

All of this accords well with what is known about the autonomic circuitry. Fibers passing without interruption from the hypothalamus to the autonomic motor neurons of the spinal cord's gray matter have recently been found, but they seem to constitute a small minority of the outgoing hypothalamic fibers; the hypothalamus has nothing like a corticospinal tract to carry its downflowing output. Instead it appears in large measure to project no farther than the midbrain, where neurons of the reticular formation take over. In fact, the pathways descending to autonomic motor neurons typically are interrupted at numerous levels. At each such interruption various further instructions can enter the descending conduction lines. It is appropriate that this should be the case. Life depends on the innervation of the viscera; in a way all the rest is biological luxury. And vital systems ought to be organized on the principle that no single excitation should greatly affect their workings. Indeed, the convergence of information on motor neurons may be as characteristic of the autonomic nervous system as it is of the somatic.

So much for the descending neural influences that ultimately act on the effector tissues of the viscera. What acts to set these influences? More specifically, what projects to the hypothalamus? Figure 2.9 shows an input that originates in a cell of the mesencephalic reticular formation, a cell whose own input derives from a fiber of the spinothalamic tract. The supposition is that in such fashion the hypothalamus may monitor the state of the internal milieu. Beyond that the search for input to the hypothalamus leads one deep into a realm of brain tissue implicated in affect and motivation, a realm in which epileptic seizures, for example, include among their signs a change in mood, sometimes to anguish or an unreasoning fear. This should not be surprising. After all, affect and motivation find observable expression in visceral and endocrine changes.

There can be little doubt, then, that the major influence exerted on the hypothalamus from the cerebral hemisphere derives from the hippocampus and the amygdala. They share this influence with few other parts of the cerebral hemisphere. For that reason a collective reference to hippocampus and amygdala is justified: they are the two principal components of what is called the limbic system. In Figure 2.9 note the presence of a two-way fiber system that curves along the edge of the neocortex from the hippocampus to the hypothalamus. The bundle is the fornix. It marks the free edge of the cerebral mantle. In both the cat and the monkey approximately two-thirds of the bundle's fibers leaving the hippocampus extend into the hypothalamus directly. The remaining third establish their synapses in the septum, from which, as the figure shows, the lines are extended, again to the hypothalamus.

We have noted that the hippocampus is a destination for sequential projections that span the neocortical sheet. It therefore becomes apparent in the tracing of visceral motor governance, as it did in the tracing of somatic, that when the tracing is done counter-current, against the direction of impulse transmission, one implicates ever greater portions of the great intermediate net. Of course, there is a difference. From a given area of neocortex, say the primary visual cortex, the road to the hippocampus must pass, with interruption, through a series of intermediate neocortical fields. The end of the neocortical road is the entorhinal area, a region of the cerebral cortex adjoining the hippocampus and intermediate in structure between it and neocortex. From here a final link completes the fiber pathways to the hippocampus. In contrast, the road to the striatum from any neocortical field whatsoever is an uninterrupted projection.

Consider next the amygdala. Although its cell architecture is quite different from that of the hippocampus, it too directs its outflow in large part to the hypothalamus. For its part the amygdala is the recipient of fibers from a district of neocortex synaptically remote from any primary sensory field. It is also, however, the recipient of fibers that originate in the olfactory cortex; indeed, so is the entorhinal area. Moreover, a part of the amygdala receives fibers from the olfactory bulb. In olfaction, therefore, the transmission of sensory data to the limbic system is remarkably direct. Why should this be so? Why should olfaction, among all the sensoria, be privileged?

One conceivable answer lies in the probability that the olfactory sensorium constitutes the earliest appearance in evolution of a capacity for sensory apprehension at a distance; it is perhaps the earliest system whereby free-ranging organisms could track sources of food and identify members of their own species and members of others. Perhaps the olfactory system, having arrived earliest, made some rather direct connections. A second conceivable answer, which does not negate the first, is that the visual recognition of an object (to take only one example) calls for complicated processing: in its highest form it requires that the arriving sensory data be made to yield a representation free from the circumstances of viewing angle, distance and illumination. How else could the object be recognized, that is, matched with past experience? Even at its simplest, say the recognition of a stripe (as by one fish viewing the flank of another) or of a moving dot (as by a frog viewing a fly), it requires the preservation well into the neural processing of topological relations in the input to the sensory sheet: the retina. Olfaction, in contrast, functions simply as a discriminator of intensity gradients. In short, olfaction as a guide to life-supporting behavior lacks much of the computational difficulty, if you will, that is inherent in vision and other sensoria.

To be sure, arguments such as these may not seem entirely convincing. If the limbic system requires of the visual, the auditory and the somatic sensoria a neocortical march, and therefore a cascading re-representation of data that originally were sensory, then why not, to an equal degree, the striatum? And why, moreover, does the striatum receive input both from the primary sensory fields and from the various association areas, in which the primary cortical data undergo successive transformations? Perhaps the heart of the difficulty is the mystery of any brain structure whose input derives, one way or another, from all (or most of) the neocortical expanse. To glibly characterize such input seems impossible, and so it is beyond us to imagine what the structure that gets it is doing with it. Yet we are presented by the central nervous system with several such structures: the limbic system, the striatum, the pons (and through it the cerebellum) and the superior colliculus.

Our survey of the mammalian central nervous system is here at its end. Its shortcomings are necessarily many. In the first place it could do little justice to the true complexity of the circuitry; if all the known systems of conduction had been mentioned, the figures in this chapter might have been rendered a hopeless tangle. For example, we left out the pons, even though that structure receives massive projections from all parts of the neocortex and sends a massive projection to the cerebellum. The lines representing those projections would have cut across several ascending and descending systems in the hindbrain.

In the second place we could make few distinctions between projections comprising millions of fibers and those comprising only a fraction of that number. It happens, for example, that the spinothalamic fibers attaining the ventral nucleus of the thalamus may number no more than a few hundred in primates, whereas the medial lemniscus has a million fibers, maybe more. Then too we could give no indication of which projections cross the midplane to the opposite side of the central nervous system and which have destinations on the same side as their origin. The central nervous system, like the rest of the body, is bilaterally symmetrical. Such distinctions play a crucial role in clinical diagnosis.

Most important, in addressing only the connectedness of the brain — that is to say, only the origins and destinations of the various fiber systems — we can evoke no more than a rough sketch of neuroanatomy: the three-dimensional architecture of the tissues stationed inside the cranium and down the core of the vertebral column. We have thereby neglected a view that has tantalized men for millenniums: the very appearance of the brain.

DEVELOPMENT AND PLASTICITY

. . .

The Development of the Brain

As the human brain develops in utero it gains neurons at the rate of hundreds of thousands a minute. One problem of neurobiology is how the neurons find their place and make the right connections.

• • •

W. Maxwell Cowan
September, 1979

The gross changes that take place during the embryonic and fetal development of the brain (see Figure 3.1) have been known for almost a century, but comparatively little is known about the underlying cellular events that give rise to the particular parts of the brain and their interconnections. What is clear is that the nervous system originates as a flat sheet of cells on the dorsal surface of the developing embryo (the neural plate), that this tissue subsequently folds into an elongated hollow structure (the neural tube) and that from the head end of the tube three prominent swellings emerge, prefiguring the three main parts of the brain (the forebrain, the midbrain and the hindbrain).

It is not on these changes in the external form of the developing brain, however, that the attention of developmental neurobiologists has focused in recent years. More interesting questions intrude. How, for instance, are the various components that constitute the major parts of the nervous system generated? How do they come to occupy their definitive locations within the brain? How do the neurons and their supporting glial cells become differentiated? How do neurons in different parts of the brain establish connections with one another? In

spite of a great deal of research effort it is still not possible to give a complete account of the development of any part of the brain, let alone of the brain as a whole. By determining what the main events in neural development are, however, one can begin to see how the critical issues are likely to be resolved.

Eight major stages can be identified in the development of any part of the brain. In the order of their appearance they are (1) the induction of the neural plate, (2) the localized proliferation of cells in different regions, (3) the migration of cells from the region in which they are generated to the places where they finally reside, (4) the aggregation of cells to form identifiable parts of the brain, (5) the differentiation of the immature neurons, (6) the formation of connections with other neurons, (7) the selective death of certain cells and (8) the elimination of some of the connections that were initially formed and the stabilization of others.

The process whereby some cells in the ectoderm, or outer layer, of the developing embryo become transformed into the specialized tissue from which the brain and spinal cord develop is called neural induction. It has been known since the 1920's that the critical event in neural induction is an interaction of the ectoderm and a part of the underlying layer of tissue called the mesoderm. The nature of this interaction remains to be elucidated, but there are good reasons for thinking that it involves the specific transfer of substances from the mesoderm to the ectoderm, and that as a result of that transfer the generalized tissue of the ectoderm becomes irreversibly committed to the formation of neural tissue. It is also clear that the sequential interaction of different parts of the ectoderm and the mesoderm results in the regional determination of the major parts of the future brain and spinal cord. The first part of the mesoderm to become associated with the ectoderm specifically induces forebrain structures, the next part leads to the formation of midbrain and hindbrain structures, and the last part to grow under the ectoderm is responsible for the later formation of the spinal cord.

Exactly how these regional determinations are brought about remains baffling. Experiments with disaggregated ectodermal and mesodermal cells from embryos of the appropriate age suggest that the critical element may be the relative concentration of two factors that are thought to be proteins with a low molecular weight. One of these, the neuralizing factor, seems to "prime" the ectoderm and to ensure its future neural character; the other, the mesodermalizing factor, appears in differing concentrations to determine the regional differences within the ectoderm.

Although a major effort was made in the 1930's and 1940's to isolate the putative inducing agents, it is clear in retrospect that much of the work was premature. Only in the past two decades has anything substantial been learned about the nature of gene induction generally, and it is still far from evident that the inductive mechanisms that have been identified in microorganisms operate in the same way in animal cells. There is another reason the problem of neural induction has proved to be so intractable. The only assay system suitable for the study of neural induction is ectoderm taken from embryos of the appropriate age, and since there is a limited period in development when the ectoderm is able to respond to the relevant inductive signals, it is necessary to work with extremely small amounts of tissue. Indeed, it is a tribute to the ingenuity and experimental skill of those who have addressed this problem that so much progress has already been made.

Once the major regions of the developing nervous system have been determined their potentialities become progressively limited as development proceeds. For example, the entire head end of the neural plate initially constitutes a forebrain-eye field from which both the forebrain and the neural part of the eye develop. If one removes a small piece of ectodermal tissue at this stage, the defect is quickly replaced by the proliferation of the neighboring cells, and the development of both the forebrain and the eye proceeds quite normally. If the same operation is done at a slightly later stage, there is a permanent defect in either the forebrain or the eye, depending on the location of the piece of tissue that was removed. In other words, at this later stage it is possible to identify a forebrain field that will give rise to definitive forebrain structures, and an eye field that will form only the neural part of the eye.

At still later stages specific regions of the forebrain become delimited within the overall forebrain field. With the aid of a variety of cell-marking techniques it has been possible to construct "fate maps" that define rather precisely the final distribution of the cells in each part of the early forebrain field (see Figure 3.2). The factors that lead to this progressive blocking out of smaller and smaller units, giving rise to specific parts of the brain, are not known, but it is not unreasonable to suppose that when more is learned about cellular differentiation in general, the problem will be clarified.

From studies of the embryos of amphibians it appears that the number of cells in the neural plate is comparatively small (on the order of 125,000) and that this number does not change much during the formation of the neural tube (see Figure 3.3). Once the neural tube has been closed off, however, cell proliferation proceeds at a brisk pace, and before long the simple layer of epithelial cells that formed the neural plate is transformed into a rather thick epithelial layer in which the cell nuclei reside at several levels. Microscopic examination of the cells, aided in some cases by the use of radioactively labeled thymidine, a specific DNA precursor, has established that all the cells in the wall of the neural tube are capable of proliferation and that the characteristic "pseudostratified" appearance of the epithelium is attributable to the fact that the nuclei of the cells are at different levels. The nuclei synthesize DNA while they lie in the depths of the epithelium, and then they migrate toward the ventricular surface and withdraw their peripheral processes before dividing. After mitosis (cell division) the daughter cells re-form their peripheral processes, and their nuclei return to the deeper part of the epithelium before reentering the mitotic

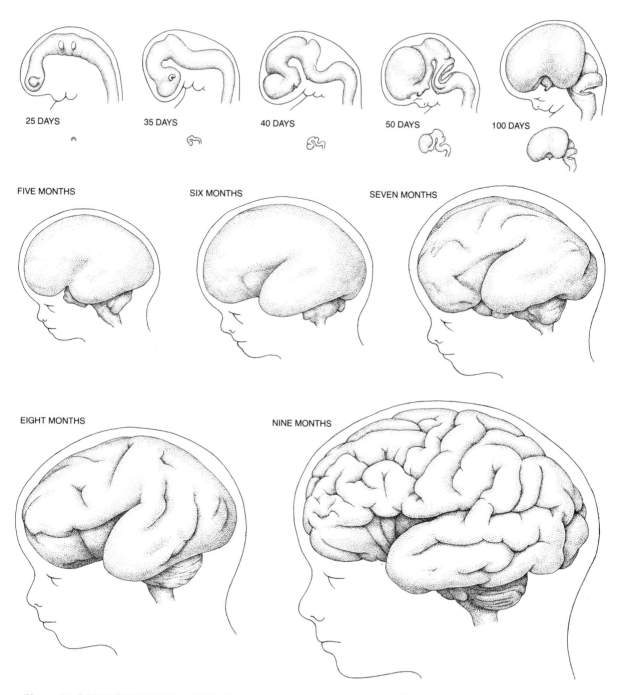

25 DAYS 35 DAYS 40 DAYS 50 DAYS 100 DAYS

FIVE MONTHS SIX MONTHS SEVEN MONTHS

EIGHT MONTHS NINE MONTHS

Figure 3.1 DEVELOPING HUMAN BRAIN viewed from the side in a succession of embryonic and fetal stages. The drawings in the main sequence (*bottom*) are reproduced at approximately four-fifths life-size. The first five embryonic stages are shown enlarged to an arbitrary common size (*top*). The forebrain, midbrain and hindbrain originate as prominent swellings at the head end of the early neural tube. In humans the cerebral hemispheres eventually overgrow the midbrain and hindbrain and partly obscure the cerebellum. The convolutions and invaginations of the brain's surface do not appear until about the middle of pregnancy. Assuming that the fully developed human brain contains 100 billion neurons and that virtually no new neurons are added after birth, neurons must be generated in the developing brain at a rate of more than 250,000 per minute.

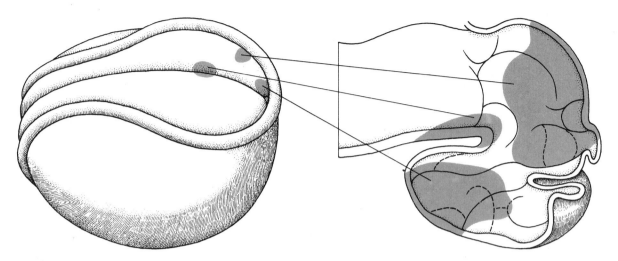

Figure 3.2 DERIVATION of each of the major regions of the brain can be traced by labeling different regions of the neural plate of an experimental animal at a very early embryonic stage with the aid of cell-marking techniques. In this demonstration of how such "fate maps" are constructed three regions have been marked on the neural plate of the early embryo of the axoloti, a large amphibian (*left*). The final positions of the cells in the marked regions are then plotted as they would be seen in a sagittal section of the brain at a later stage of embryonic development (*right*). This illustration is adapted from the work of D. C.-O. Jacobson of the University of Uppsala.

cycle. The migration of the nuclei of proliferating neurons is characteristic of epithelial cells of this kind (see Figure 3.4).

After the cells pass through a number of such cycles (the number varies from region to region and from population to population within any one region), they apparently lose their capacity for synthesizing DNA, and they migrate out of the epithelium to form a second cellular layer adjacent to the ventricular zone. The cells that constitute this mantle, or intermediate, layer are young neurons, which never again divide, and glial-cell precursors, which retain their capacity for proliferation throughout life.

Although it is not known what turns the proliferative mechanism on and off in any region of the nervous system, it is clear that the relative times at which different populations of cells cease dividing is rigidly determined, and there is now a sizable body of evidence to suggest that this is a critical stage in the life of all neurons. Not only does the withdrawal of a cell from the mitotic cycle seem to trigger its subsequent migration into the intermediate layer but also the cell seems at the same time to acquire a definitive "address," in the sense that if its "birth date" (defined as the time when a cell loses its capacity for DNA synthesis) is known, it is possible to predict where the cell will finally reside.

Furthermore, it seems in some cases that the pattern of connections the neuron will ultimately form is also determined at this time.

From experiments in which small amounts of radioactively labeled thymidine have been administered to embryos (or in the case of mammals to their pregnant mothers) investigators now know the birth dates of the cells in many parts of the brain for a number of different species. From these studies it is now possible to make several generalizations about the patterning of cell proliferation in the brain. First, the larger neurons, including most of the cells whose processes extend for considerable distances, such as the cells in the retina that project to the visual centers of the brain, are usually generated earlier than the smaller neurons, whose fibers are confined to the region of the cell body. Second, the sequence of cell proliferation is characteristic for each region of the brain. For example, in the cerebral cortex the first cells to withdraw from the proliferative cycle will in time come to occupy the deepest cortical layer, whereas those that are generated at successively later times form the progressively more superficial layers of the cortex (see Figure 3.5).

On the other hand, in the neural retina (which is actually an extension of the brain) the sequence of

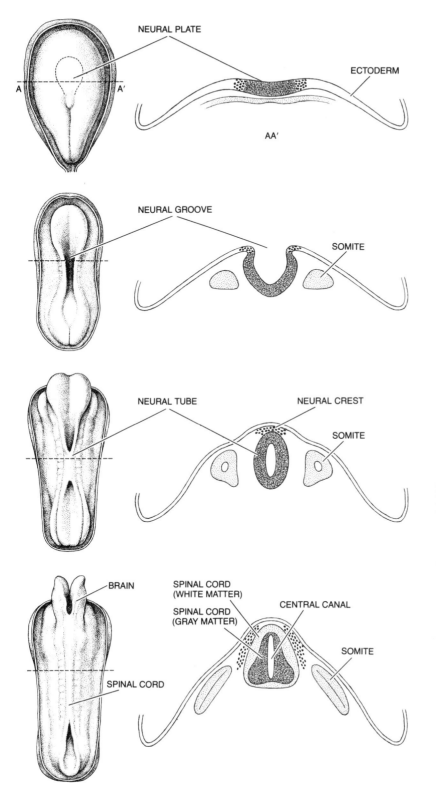

NEURAL PLATE

ECTODERM

AA′

NEURAL GROOVE

SOMITE

NEURAL TUBE

NEURAL CREST

SOMITE

BRAIN

SPINAL CORD
(WHITE MATTER)

SPINAL CORD
(GRAY MATTER)

CENTRAL CANAL

SOMITE

SPINAL CORD

Figure 3.3 GENESIS OF THE NERVOUS SYSTEM from the ectoderm of a human embryo during the third and fourth weeks after conception is represented in these drawings, which show both an external view of the developing embryo (*left*) and a corresponding cross-sectional view at about the middle of the future spinal cord (*right*). The central nervous system begins as the neural plate, a flat sheet of ectodermal cells on the dorsal surface of the embryo that folds into a hollow structure called the neural tube. The head end of the central canal widens to form the ventricles, or cavities, of the brain. The peripheral nervous system is derived largely from the cells of the neural crest and from motor-nerve fibers that leave the lower part of the brain at each segment of the future spinal cord.

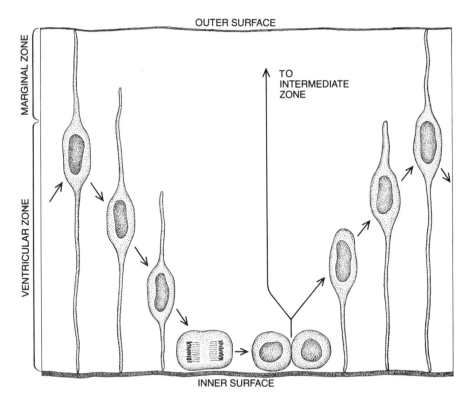

Figure 3.4 NUCLEI OF NERVE CELLS MIGRATE in the layer of epithelial tissue that forms the wall of the neural tube in the developing embryo. When the cells in this layer, called the neuroepithelium or ventricular zone, replicate their DNA, their nuclei migrate toward the inner surface of the epithelium, their peripheral processes become detached from the outermost layer and the cells become rounded before dividing. After mitosis (cell division) the daughter cells either extend a new process so that their nuclei can migrate back to the middle level of the epithelium, or (if the cells have stopped dividing) they migrate out of the epithelium to form part of the intermediate zone in the wall of the brain.

cell proliferation is essentially the reverse; the first population of cells to be generated (the ganglion cells) migrates to the most superficial layer of the retina, and subsequent populations of cells occupy progressively deeper layers. In other regions of the brain the sequences are more complex, but in each region it is evident that cells occupying similar positions are always generated at the same time; conversely, cells generated at different times invariably come to reside in different zones within the region. A third generalization that can be made is that in most parts of the brain the first supporting cells to be formed appear at about the same time as the first neurons, but as a rule the proliferation of glial cells continues for a much longer period.

The number of neurons initially formed in any region of the brain is determined by three factors.

The first factor is the duration of the proliferative period as a whole; in the regions that have been studied to date, it has been found to range from a few days to several weeks. The second factor is the duration of the cell cycle; in young embryos it is usually on the order of a few hours, but as development progresses it may become as long as four or five days. The third factor is the number of precursor cells from which the neuronal population is derived.

A number of methods are now available for determining the duration of the proliferative period and the length of the cell cycle, but except in a few cases it is not possible to estimate the size of the precursor pool of cells. Part of the reason for this difficulty is that it is impossible at present to follow the fate of individual cells in the developing mammalian brain, as has been done in the much simpler nervous systems of certain invertebrates. In these organisms the embryos are often quite transparent, and individual cells can be followed through several mitotic divisions with the aid of a light microscope equipped with differential-interference optics. Alternatively, the precursor cells in such organisms may be so large that they can be readily labeled by the intracellular injection of marker molecules such as horseradish peroxidase; if the marker is not degraded, it can be distributed to all the cell's progeny, at least over several cell generations.

S ince most neurons are generated in or close to the ventricular lining of the neural tube and finally come to rest at some distance from this layer, they have to go through at least one phase of migration after withdrawing from the proliferative cycle.

There are a few situations in which cells migrate away from the ventricular zone but continue to proliferate. This is usually observed in a special region found between the ventricular and the intermediate zone, known as the subventricular zone. This layer, which is particularly prominent in the forebrain, gives rise to many of the smaller neurons in some of the deep structures of the cerebral hemisphere (the basal ganglia), to certain small cortical neurons and to many of the glial cells in the cerebral cortex and the underlying white matter. In the hindbrain some of the cells in the corresponding subventricular region undergo a second migration under the surface of the developing cerebellum, where they set up a special proliferative zone known as the external granular layer. In the human brain proliferation in this layer continues for several weeks and gives rise to most of the interneurons in the cerebellar cortex,

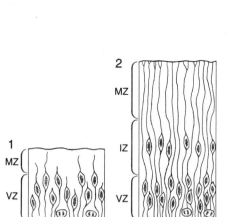
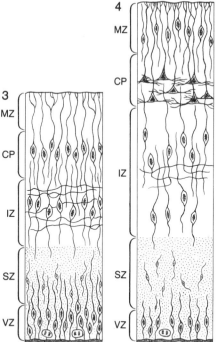

Figure 3.5 THE WALL OF THE DEVELOPING BRAIN at the earliest stage (1) consists only of a "pseudostratified" epithelium, in which the ventricular zone (*VZ*) contains the cell bodies and the marginal zone (*MZ*) contains only the extended outer cell processes. When some of the cells lose their capacity for synthesizing DNA and withdraw from the mitotic cycle (2), they form the intermediate zone (*IZ*). In the forebrain the cells that pass through this zone aggregate to form the cortical plate (*CP*), the region in which the various layers of the cerebral cortex develop (3). At the latest stage (4) the original ventricular zone remains as the ependymal lining of the cerebral ventricles, and the comparatively cell-free region between this lining and the cortex becomes the subcortical white matter. Subventricular zone (*SZ*) is a second proliferative region in which many glial cells and some neurons are generated.

including the billions of granule cells that are a distinctive feature of the cerebellum. With these and a few other exceptions, most migrations of neurons involve the movement of postmitotic cells.

The process of neuronal migration appears in most cases to be amoeboid. The migrating cells extend a leading process that attaches itself to some appropriate substrate; the nucleus flows or is drawn into the process, and the trailing process behind the nucleus is then withdrawn. It is a fairly slow procedure, the average rate of migration being on the order of a tenth of a millimeter per day. In a few cases the cell as a whole does not migrate. Instead it begins to form some of its processes at an early stage in its development, and later the cell body begins to move progressively farther away from the first processes, which remain essentially where they originated.

Since neurons often migrate over considerable distances, it would be interesting to know to what types of directional cue they respond. In particular, how do they know when to stop migrating and to begin aggregating with other neurons of the same kind? It has been known for some time that there are specialized glial cells within the developing brain whose cell bodies lie inside the ventricular zone and whose processes extend radially to the surface (see Figure 3.6). Since these cells appear at an early stage of development and persist until some time after neuronal migration has ceased, it has been suggested that they might provide an appropriate scaffolding along which the migrating neurons might move. Certainly in electron micrographs of most parts of the developing brain the migrating cells are almost invariably found to be closely associated with the neighboring glial processes, as shown in Figure 3.7. This relation has led Pasko Rakic of the Yale University School of Medicine to postulate that migrating cells are directed to their definitive locations by such glial processes. In support of this view Rakic and Richard L. Sidman of the Children's Hospital Medical Center in Boston have noted that in one of the most striking genetic mutations affecting the cerebellum of the mouse the radial glial processes degenerate at a comparatively early stage; apparently as a result of this degeneration the migration of most of the granule cells is severely disrupted.

Considering the distances over which many neurons move in the course of development, it is perhaps not surprising that during their migration some cells are misdirected and end up in distinctly abnormal positions. Such neuronal misplacements (termed ectopias) have long been recognized by pathologists as a concomitant of certain gross disorders in brain development, but it is not generally appreciated that even during normal development a proportion of the migrating cells may respond inappropriately to the usual directional cues and end up in aberrant locations. Recent technical advances have made it possible to recognize cells of this kind in several situations, and it is significant that the majority of such misplaced neurons appear to be eliminated during the later stages of development. In one population of neurons that has been carefully studied from this point of view, about 3 percent of the cells have been found to migrate to some abnormal location; all but a handful of these misplaced neurons, however, degenerate during the later phase of naturally occurring cell death.

When the migrating neurons reach their definitive locations, they generally aggregate with other cells of a similar kind to form either cortical layers or nuclear masses. The tendency of developing cells of the same embryonic origin to selectively adhere to one another was first demonstrated more than 50 years ago, but it is only in the past decade that this subject has attracted the attention it deserves from neuroembryologists. Much of the initial stimulus for the more recent work stemmed from the search for the molecular mechanisms underlying the formation of specific connections between related groups of neurons. Unfortunately that problem has proved to be intractable, but much of the work that was done on it bears directly on the important issue of how discrete populations of neurons are formed in the developing brain.

Perhaps the most important finding to come out of these studies is that when cells from two or three regions of the developing nervous system are dissociated (usually mechanically or by mild chemical treatment), mixed together and then allowed to reaggregate in an appropriate medium, they tend to sort themselves out so that the cells from each region preferentially aggregate with other cells from the same region. This selective adhesiveness seems to be a general property of all living cells and is probably due to the appearance on their surfaces of specific classes of large molecules that serve both to "recognize" cells of the same kind and to bind the cells together. These molecules, which function as ligands between cells, appear to be highly specific for each major type of cell. Moreover, they appear to change in either number or distribution as devel-

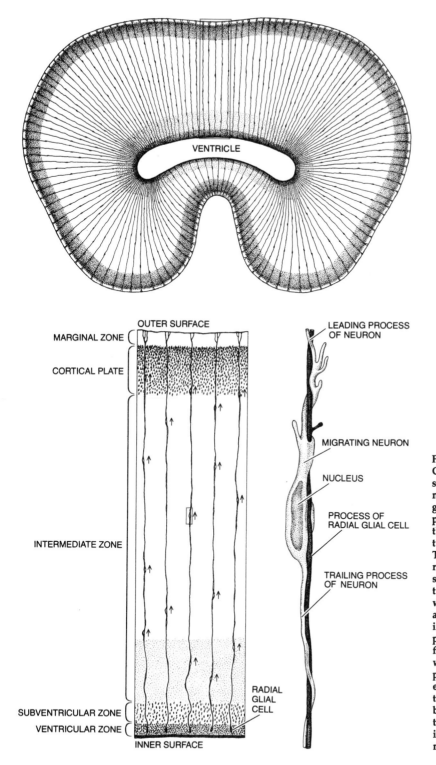

Figure 3.6 **RADIAL GLIAL CELLS** arise during the early stages of the development of the nervous system and are distinguished by their extremely long processes, which span the entire thickness of the wall of the neural tube and its derivative structures. The top drawing shows how the radial glial cells look in a Golgi-stained preparation of a thick transverse section through the wall of the cerebral hemisphere of a fetal monkey. The cell bodies lie in the ventricular zone and their processes extend to the outer surface of the surrounding layers, where they appear to form expanded terminal attachments. An enlarged view of a segment of this transverse section is shown at the bottom left. The small portion of tissue inside the colored rectangle in this enlargement is further magnified at the bottom right.

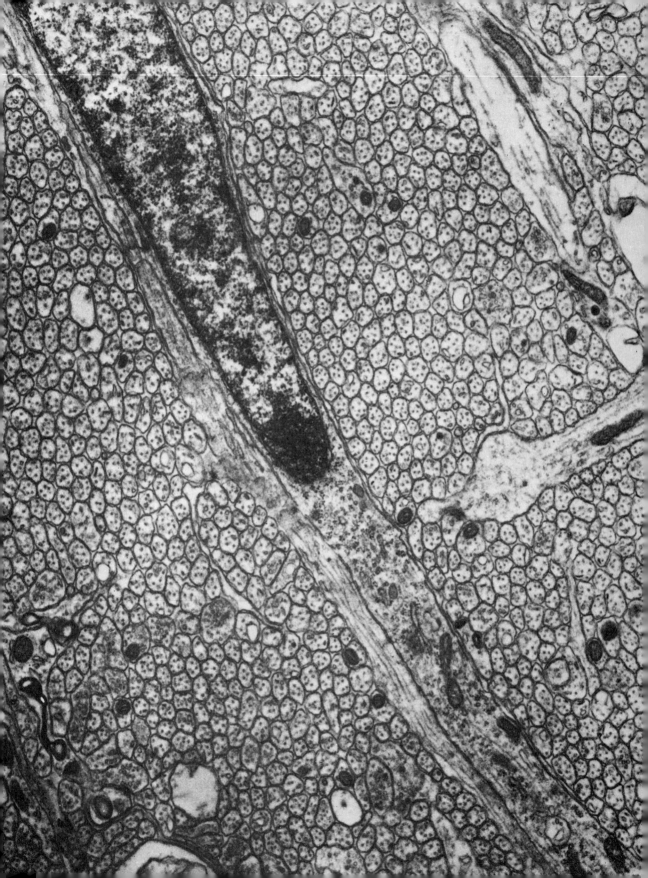

Figure 3.7 MIGRATION OF A YOUNG NEURON from its birthplace deep in the cerebellum of a fetal monkey toward the outer surface of the developing brain is captured in this micrograph by Pasko Rakic of the Yale University School of Medicine. The migrating neuron is the broader of the two diagonal bands running from the top left to the bottom right; the dark, oblong object inside the upper part of this band is the nucleus of the nerve cell. The lighter, narrower band along the underside of the neuron is the elongated process of a glial cell, which serves both as a supporting structure and as a guide for the migrating neuron. The neuron travels through a dense neuropile, or feltwork of nerve fibers, which run in various directions. Although the migrating neuron is in contact with thousands of other cellular processes, it remains intimately associated with the glial cell along its entire length. This section of brain tissue is magnified about 22,000 diameters.

opment proceeds. At present workers in several laboratories are endeavoring to isolate and characterize these and other surface ligands, and it seems likely that this may be the first major problem in neural development to be successfully analyzed at the molecular level.

One special feature of cell aggregation in the developing nervous system is that in most regions of the brain the cells not only adhere to one another but also adopt some preferential orientation. For example, in the cerebral cortex the majority of the large pyramidal neurons are consistently aligned with their prominent apical dendrites directed toward the surface and their axons directed toward the underlying white matter. It is not evident how cells come to be aligned in this way, but it seems likely that it is attributable either to the existence of different classes of cell-surface molecules specifically concerned with cell-cell orientation or to the selective redistribution of surface molecules responsible for the cell's initial aggregation.

One of the most striking features in the development of neurons is the progressive elaboration of their processes, but this is only one aspect of their differentiation. Equally important are their adoption of a particular mode of transmission (most neurons generate action potentials but some show only decremental transmission) and the selection of one or the other of two modes of interaction with other cells (either by the formation of conventional synapses to provide for the release of a chemical transmitter or by the formation of gap junctions to provide for electrical interactions of cells). Neurobi-

ologists are only now beginning to learn something of these more covert aspects of neuronal differentiation, and it is becoming clear that neurons may be considerably more complex than had been imagined. For example, it has recently been shown that some neurons can switch from one chemical transmitter to another (specifically from norepinephrine to acetylcholine) under the influence of certain environmental factors, whereas others can show a change in the principal ion they use for the propagation of nerve impulses at different developmental stages (changing, for instance, from calcium to sodium).

Rather more is known about the formation of neuronal processes. Most neurons in the brain of mammals are multipolar, with several tapering dendrites, which generally function as receptive processes, and a single axon, which serves as the cell's main effector process. Although some cells are known to form processes before they start migrating, the majority begin to generate processes only after reaching their final position. Exactly what stimulates the formation of processes is not clear. Studies in which immature neurons have been isolated and maintained in tissue culture reveal that processes are formed only when the cells are able to adhere to an appropriate substrate and that under these conditions the cells are often able to form a fairly normal complement of both dendrites and axons. In some cases, in spite of the highly artificial conditions in which the neurons are grown, the overall appearance of the dendrites that are formed closely resembles that seen in the intact brain, even though the cells are deprived of all contact with other neurons or even glial cells. Observations of this kind suggest that the information required for a neuron to generate its distinctive dendritic branching is genetically determined.

It is also evident, however, that during the normal development of the brain most neurons are subject to a variety of local mechanical influences that may modify their form. Certainly the number and distribution of the inputs the cells receive may critically affect their final shape. A striking example of this effect is seen in the cerebellum. The dendrites of the most distinctive class of neurons in the cerebellar cortex, the Purkinje cells, normally have a characteristic planar arrangement that is oriented at right angles to the axons of the granule cells that constitute their principal input; if for any reason the usual regular arrangement of the granule cells' axons is disrupted, the planar distribution of the dendrites of the Purkinje cells is correspondingly altered.

The actual mechanism by which the processes of a neuron are elongated is now quite well understood. Most processes bear distinctive structures at their growing ends called growth cones (see Figure 3.8). These expanded, highly motile structures, which in the living state seem to be continually exploring their immediate environment, are the sites where most new material is added to the growing process. When a process branches, it almost always does so by the formation of a new growth cone. Although the evidence is largely indirect, there are reasons for thinking the growth cone has encoded within (or on) it the necessary molecular features that enable it both to detect appropriate substrates along which to grow and to identify appropriate targets. Experiments in which neurons have been grown on a variety of artificial substrates indicate that most processes grow preferentially along surfaces of high adhesiveness.

One of the least well understood problems in the entire field of developmental neurobiology is how axons are able to find their way. It is particularly difficult to see how they do so when they may have to extend for considerable distances within the brain and at one or more points along their course deviate either to the right or to the left, cross to the opposite side of the brain and give off one or more branches before finally reaching their predetermined destination. In some systems it looks as if the axons simply grow under the influence of certain gradients that act along the major axes of the brain and spinal cord; in other systems the axons seem to be guided by their relation to their nearest neighbors. In many cases, however, it appears that the growing axon has encoded within it a sophisticated molecular mechanism that enables it to correctly respond to structural or chemical cues along its route.

Such directionally guided growth has recently

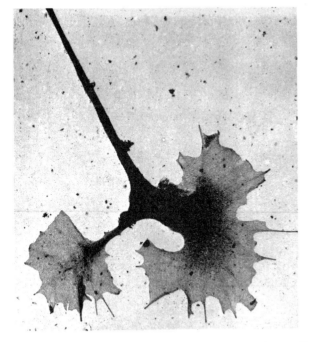 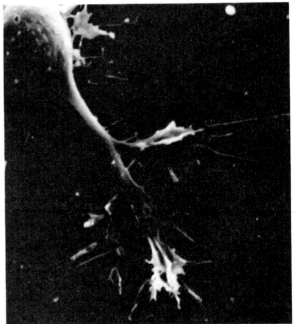

Figure 3.8 GROWTH CONES are expanded, highly motile structures found at the ends of growing neuronal processes. The micrograph at the left (made by J. Michael Cochran and Mary Bartlett Bunge) shows a pair of growth cones at the end of an axonlike process of a sympathetic ganglion cell from a rat. The cell had been dissociated and grown in tissue culture, and the process seen here had branched just a few minutes before the cell was fixed and prepared (without sectioning) for viewing. The fine, fingerlike extensions are filopodia; the flattened veil-like sheets between them are lamellipodia. The micrograph at the right (by Steven R. Rothman) shows a growing dendrite of a neuron obtained from the hippocampus of a fetal rat's brain. The growth cones were formed after the neuron had been dissociated and grown in tissue culture for only two hours.

been demonstrated by Rita Levi-Montalcini of the Laboratory of Cell Biology of the National Research Council in Rome. When she and her colleagues injected the protein known as nerve-growth factor into the brain of young rats, there was an abnormal growth of axons from sympathetic ganglion cells (peripheral neurons that lie alongside the vertebral column and are known to be sensitive to nerve-growth factor) into the spinal cord and up toward the brain, apparently along the route of diffusion of the injected nerve-growth factor. In this case the nerve-growth factor was acting not so much as a trophic, or growth-promoting, substance (as it usually does) but rather as a tropic, or direction-determining, substance, and the sympathetic nerve axons were responding chemotropically to its presence.

There are two other features of the growth of nerve processes that merit comment. The first is that most neurons seem to generate many more processes than are needed or than they are subsequently able to maintain. Hence most young neurons bear large numbers of short dendritelike processes, all but a few of which are later retracted as the cells mature. Similarly, most developing axons appear to make many more connections than are needed in the mature state, and commonly there is a phase of process elimination during which many (and in some cases all but one) of the initial group of connections are withdrawn. The second feature is that there is a strong tendency for axons to grow in close association with their neighbors, a phenomenon known as fasciculation. Recent work suggests that the tendency to fasciculate may be associated with the appearance along the length of most axons of surface ligands that enable them to join up and grow with other axons of a similar kind. In at least one instance it seems that because of this type of lateral association only the first axon in the group needs to develop a conventional growth cone; the other axons simply follow the leader.

U ndoubtedly the most important unresolved issue in the development of the brain is the question of how neurons make specific patterns of connections. Earlier notions that most of the connectivity of the brain was functionally selected from a randomly generated set of connections are now seen to be untenable. Most of the connections seem to be precisely established at an early stage of development, and there is much evidence that the connections formed are specific not only for particular regions of the brain but also for particular neurons

(and in some cases particular parts of the neurons) within these regions.

Several hypotheses have been put forward to explain how this remarkable precision is brought about. Some workers have argued that it can be simply explained on the basis that growing axons maintain the same topographical relation to one another as their parent cell bodies have. Others have suggested that the timing of events (in particular the time at which different groups of fibers reach their target regions) is critical. The one explanation that seems to fit all the observed phenomena is the chemoaffinity hypothesis, first formulated by Roger W. Sperry of the California Institute of Technology. According to this view most neurons (or more likely most small populations of neurons) become chemically differentiated at an early stage in their development depending on the positions they occupy, and this aspect of their differentiation is expressed in the form of distinguishing labels that enable the axons of the neurons to recognize either a matching label or a complementary one on the surface of their target neurons.

Although the problem is a general one affecting all parts of the nervous system, it has been most intensively studied in two systems: the innervation of the limb musculature by the relevant motor neurons in the spinal cord and the projection of the ganglion cells in the retina of the eye to their principal terminus in the brain of lower vertebrates, the optic tectum. Studies of muscle innervation indicate that under normal circumstances small populations of motor neurons, called motor-neuron pools, become segregated at an early stage in development, and that each motor-neuron pool preferentially innervates a specific limb muscle, few errors being made in the process. Although the specificity of the innervation pattern is normally precise, it is not absolute. Hence if a supernumerary hindlimb from a donor chick embryo is transplanted alongside the normal hindlimb of a host embryo, the muscles in the supernumerary limb invariably become innervated by motor-neuron pools that normally innervate either parts of the trunk or the limb-girdle musculature. The pattern of innervation is clearly aberrant, but the fact that the muscles in the transplanted limb are always innervated by the same populations of cells strongly suggests that even under these unusual conditions the axons of the motor neurons obey some (as yet unidentified) set of rules.

The retinotectal system has proved to be particularly advantageous for the analysis of the problem. In amphibians it is possible at the embryonic and larval stages to carry out a variety of experimental manipulations such as rotating the eye, making compound eyes with pieces of tissue obtained from different segments of two or more retinas and ablating or rotating parts of the tectum (see Figure 3.9). Later, when the system is fully developed, it is quite easy to determine the connections formed by the retinal ganglion cells anatomically, electrophysiologically or behaviorally. Furthermore, in fishes and amphibians the optic nerve (which is formed by the axons of the retinal ganglion cells) is capable of regeneration after its fibers have been interrupted, so that it is possible to carry out many of the same kinds of experimental manipulation in juvenile or adult animals. Since there is now a vast body of literature on this system, only some of the major findings can be summarized here.

Perhaps the most important findings to have emerged from this work come from two main groups of experiments. In the first group of experiments an optic nerve was cut in frogs and salamanders, and the eye was rotated through 180 degrees. In the other experiments portions of the optic tectum of goldfish and frogs were excised and the excised portions were either rotated or transferred to another part of the tectum. In both groups of experiments the regenerating fibers of the optic nerve could be shown, either electrophysiologically or behaviorally, to have grown back to the same parts of the tectum as those they originally innervated. The simplest explanation for this finding is that the axons of the ganglion cells and their target neurons in the optic tectum are labeled in some way, and that the regenerating axons grow back until they "recognize" the appropriate labels on the neurons in the relevant part of the optic tectum.

It is difficult to refute the argument that under such circumstances the fibers from different parts of the retina had earlier "imprinted" themselves on the related groups of tectal cells, and that the axons or the tectal neurons simply "remembered" their previous position. There is some evidence to suggest, however, that a similar mechanism may account for the initial development of the system. If the developing eye of a frog is rotated before a certain critical stage in development, the resulting projection of the retina on the tectum tends to be normal. If the rotation is done after the critical period, however, the retinal projection is invariably rotated to the same degree. Similarly, if the entire embryonic optic tectum is rotated by 180 degrees in the head-to-tail dimension (together with a portion of the forebrain that lies just in front of it), the retinal projection that is formed is again inverted.

These experiments suggest that there is a certain stage in the development of most neural centers during which they become topographically polarized in such a way that the constituent neurons acquire some determining characteristic that establishes the spatial organization of the projection as a whole. Marcus Jacobson of the University of Miami School of Medicine showed some years ago that in the clawed frog *Xenopus laevis* the retina becomes polarized in this way at about the time the first ganglion cells withdraw from the mitotic cycle. Although at this stage only about 1 percent of the ganglion cells are present, the entire future patterning of the retinal projection on the tectum seems to be established at the same time. It is not at all clear how neurons acquire positional information of this type or how it is expressed in the outgrowth of their processes. It appears, however, that the polarity-determining mechanisms are not confined to the nervous system but operate throughout the organism. R. Kevin Hunt of Johns Hopkins University and Jacobson have found that if a developing eye is transplanted into the flank of a larval frog before the period of axial specification and allowed to pass through the critical period in this abnormal position, then when it is retransplanted into the orbit, or eye socket, the ganglion cells form connections within the optic tectum that reflect the orientation of the eye during the period it was in the flank, rather than its position after it was replaced in the orbit.

When a growing axon reaches its appropriate target, whether it is another group of neurons or an effector tissue such as a collection of muscle or gland cells, it forms specialized functional contacts —synapses— with these cells. It is at such sites that information is transmitted from one cell to another, usually through the release of small quantities of an appropriate transmitter [see "The Chemistry of the Brain," by Leslie L. Iversen; SCIENTIFIC AMERICAN, September, 1979; Offprint 1441]. A large body of nomenological evidence suggests that at synapses there is an important two-way transfer of substances essential for the survival and normal functioning of both the presynaptic and the postsynaptic cells. These substances, which are collectively referred to as trophic factors, are for the most part hypothetical; only one (nerve-growth factor) has

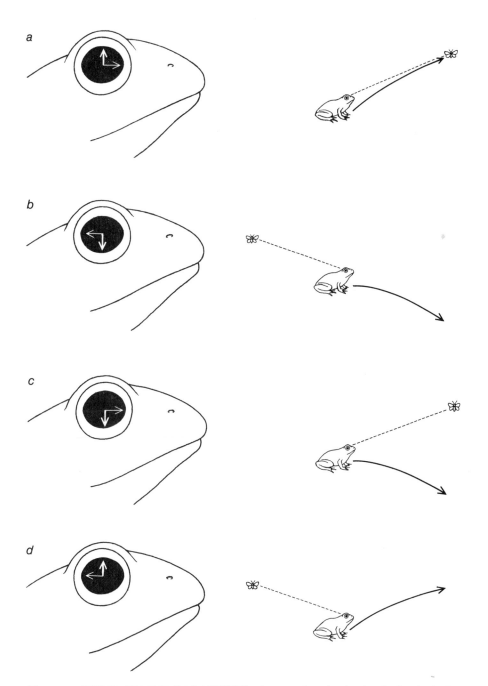

Figure 3.9 STUDY OF NEURON PATTERNS of connections in the developing brain involves manipulating the projection of the retina on the optic tectum of the midbrain. Drawing *a* shows the behavior of a control frog with its eyes in the normal positions. In experiment *b* the right eye had been rotated through 180 degrees; when the frog was tested after the optic nerve had regenerated, the frog's attempt to strike at a lure placed in its upper field of view was exactly 180 degrees in the wrong direction. In experiment *c* the left eye was substituted for the right, inverting only the dorsoventral axis (*thick arrow*); the frog directed its strike forward toward the lure, but in the direction of the lower visual field. In experiment *d* a similar transplantation was done, but this time inverting the eye only in the anteroposterior direction (*thin arrow*); the frog sensed that the lure was in the upper visual field, but it now struck forward instead of backward.

been identified and chemically characterized. This substance, which was first identified by Viktor Hamburger and Levi-Montalcini at Washington University in the 1950's, has been found to be a protein that normally exists in the form of a pair of identical amino acid chains, each with a molecular weight of slightly more than 13,000 daltons.

Although the mode of action of nerve-growth factor has not yet been defined, it is known to be essential for the growth and survival of sympathetic ganglion cells, and during development it specifically promotes the outgrowth of processes from these and from certain spinal ganglion cells. In addition, as I have already noted, in some cases it may influence the directed outgrowth of sympathetic nerve fibers. Conversely, if an antibody to nerve-growth factor is administered to newborn mice, it leads to the destruction of the entire sympathetic nervous system. Even in adult animals nerve-growth factor appears to be continually supplied to sympathetic neurons by their target tissues, the protein being taken up by the terminal portions of their axons and transported back to the cell body. If the supply is interrupted by cutting the axons of the sympathetic neurons, their functional integrity is seriously disturbed and the synapses that end on the cells are promptly withdrawn. It seems probable that in the next few years several other substances of this kind will be isolated, and it may well be shown that most classes of neurons are dependent on a specific agent for their survival and for the directed growth of their processes.

It has become evident in recent years that the development of many structures and tissues is sculptured by highly programmed phases of cell death. This is true also of the developing brain. In many regions of the brain the number of neurons originally generated greatly exceeds the number of neurons that survive beyond the developmental period. In each region for which quantitative data are available it has been found that the number of neurons is adjusted during a phase of selective cell death that always occupies a predictable period (usually at about the time when the population of neurons as a whole is forming synaptic connections with its target tissue). It is not known whether this phenomenon operates in every part of the brain (it has been studied mainly in small groups of cells), but in those where it has been documented it in-

volves between 15 and 85 percent of the initial neuronal population.

It seems, therefore, that in many parts of the brain the final size of the neuronal population is established in two stages: an early stage in which a comparatively large number of cells are generated, and a later stage in which the number of neurons is adjusted to match the size of the field they innervate. It is commonly assumed that the limiting factor determining the final number of cells is the number of functional contacts available to the axons of the developing neurons. Certainly if one experimentally reduces the size of the projection field, the magnitude of the naturally occurring cell death is accentuated to a proportional degree. In the case of the spinal motor neurons that innervate the hindlimb musculature it has been possible to reduce the amount of cell death in chick embryos by experimentally adding a supernumerary limb. Recent experiments suggest, however, that it may not be the formation of connections that is critical but rather the amount of trophic material available to the cells.

At a somewhat later stage in development there is a second adjustment, not in the size of the neuronal population as a whole but in the number of processes its cells maintain. The phenomenon of process (and synapse) elimination was first observed in the innervation of the limb muscles in young rats. Whereas in mature animals most muscle cells are innervated by a single axon, during the first postnatal week as many as five or six separate axons can be shown to form synapses with each muscle fiber. Over the course of the next two or three weeks the additional axons are successively eliminated, until only one axon survives. A comparable phase of process elimination has also been found in certain neuron-to-neuron connections both in the peripheral nervous system and in the brain. To cite just one example, in the cerebellum of adult animals each Purkinje cell receives only a single incoming nerve fiber of the class known as climbing fibers, but during the immediate postnatal period several such fibers may contact each Purkinje cell. Except in certain genetic mutations that affect the cerebellum all but one of these fibers are eliminated.

The finding that many early processes are later eliminated raises an interesting question: What determines which processes survive and which are eliminated? At present one can only surmise that during development fibers compete among themselves in some way. There is evidence to suggest that one factor that may give some fibers a competitive edge over the others is their functional activity. Certainly in many systems the final form of the relevant neuronal populations emerges only gradually from a rather amorphous structure, and it is often possible to alter markedly the final appearance of the structure and its connections by interfering with its function during certain critical periods in its development. Two examples drawn from the sensory areas of the cerebral cortex will serve to make this point.

In the macaque monkey information from the retina reaches the fourth layer of the visual cortex by way of a structure called the lateral geniculate nucleus. At this level in the cortex the inputs from the two eyes are quite separate, a fact that has been directly demonstrated in experimental animals by injecting large amounts of a radioactively labeled amino acid into one eye. The retinal ganglion cells take up the labeled amino acid, incorporate it into protein and transport it to the lateral geniculate nucleus. Here some fraction of the label is released and becomes available for incorporation by the geniculate cells, which can then transport it along their axons to the visual cortex. In suitably prepared autoradiographs (in which the distribution of the labeled fibers reaching the cortex can be visualized) it is evident that the primary visual area is arranged into alternating eye-dominance bands, each band about 400 micrometers wide, that receive their input from either the right eye or the left eye. David H. Hubel, Torsten N. Wiesel and Simon LeVay showed that if the eyelids of one eye of an experimental animal are sutured shut shortly after birth (so that the retina of the eye is never exposed to patterned illumination), the eye-dominance bands connected to the deprived eye are much narrower than normal bands. At the same time the bands connected with the open eye are correspondingly wider (the overall width of two adjoining bands remaining constant).

This result appears to be brought about partly by the shrinkage of the eye-dominance bands connected to the deprived eye, accompanied by a secondary expansion of those associated with the nondeprived, normal eye, and partly by the persistence of an earlier, more widespread distribution of the fibers from the nondeprived eye. If the inputs from the two eyes are examined at diffrent stages in development, it can be shown that when the fibers from the lateral geniculate nucleus first reach the visual cortex, the inputs from one eye extensively overlap those from the other. It is not until about the end of the first postnatal month that the eye-dominance bands become clearly defined. In the light of this discovery (and the results of experiments in which the deprived eye is reopened and the other eye is sutured shut) it seems likely that the effect of visual deprivation is to place geniculocortical cells that are connected with a deprived eye at some disadvantage, so that they become less effective in competing for synaptic sites on the target cells in the fourth layer of the cortex.

In the corresponding layer in the sensory cortex of the mouse the cells are arranged in a number of distinctive groupings called barrels (see Figure 3.10). Physiological studies have shown that each barrel receives its input from a single whisker on the opposite side of the mouse's snout, the whiskers being among the most important sense organs in mice. Thomas A. Woolsey of the Washington University School of Medicine, who first recognized the importance of the barrels, has found that if a small group of whiskers is removed during the first few days after birth, the corresponding group of barrels in the cortex fails to develop. This is a particularly interesting finding because there are at least two intervening groups of neurons between the sensory neurons that innervate the whiskers and the neurons that constitute the cortical barrels.

These and many other observations make it clear that the developing brain is an extremely plastic structure. Although many regions may be "hardwired," others (such as the cerebral cortex) are open to a variety of influences, both intrinsic and environmental. The ability of the brain to reorganize itself in response to external influences or to localized injury is currently one of the most active areas in neurobiological research, not only because of its obvious relevance for such phenomena as learning and memory, and its bearing on the capacity of the brain to recover after injury, but also because of what it is likely to reveal about normal brain development.

Finally, it is worth pointing out that the development of the brain, like the development of most other biological structures, is not without error. I have already indicated that errors may appear during neuronal migration. There are also several known cases in which errors are made during the formation of connections. In the visual system it has

a

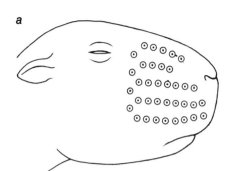

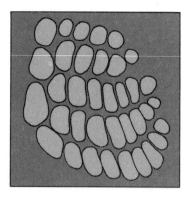

b

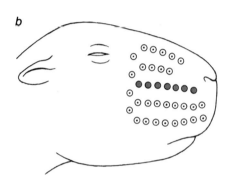

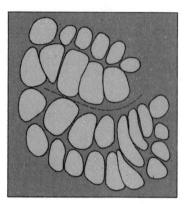

Figure 3.10 **WHISKERS AND BARRELS** in a young mouse are one of many systems that have been found to demonstrate the critical dependence of the developing nervous system on its inputs. The whiskers in this case are the sensory hairs on a mouse's snout; the barrels are specialized aggregations of neurons in the fourth layer of the mouse's cerebral cortex. Each barrel receives its input from a single whisker on the opposite side of the mouse's snout (*a*). If one row of whiskers is destroyed shortly after birth, the corresponding row of barrels in the cerebral cortex will later be found to be missing and the adjoining barrels to be enlarged (*b, c*). If all the whiskers are destroyed, the entire group of barrels will have disappeared (*d*). The figure is based on work of Thomas A. Woolsey of Washington University School of Medicine.

c

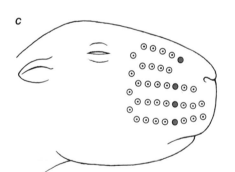

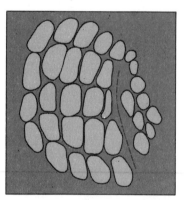

d

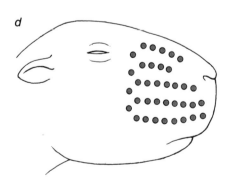

been noted by a number of workers that some optic-nerve fibers that should cross the midline in the optic chiasm grow back aberrantly to the same side of the brain. In some of these situations if one eye is removed from an experimental animal early in development, the number of aberrantly directed fibers can be considerably increased. Since such aberrant fibers are often not seen in the mature brain, it looks as if the misdirected axons (and what-ever inappropriate connections they form) are eliminated at later stages in development. How they are recognized as being erroneous and how they are subsequently removed remains a puzzle. Considering the complexity of the developmental mechanisms involved, it is hardly surprising that errors are found. What is surprising is that they appear infrequently and that they are often effectively eliminated.

The Development of Maps and Stripes in the Brain

In the human brain nerve cells form maps of their relations with the external world, and the maps are divided into stripes. How the stripes form is explored by creating a frog with three eyes.

. . .

Martha Constantine-Paton and Margaret I. Law
December, 1982

The brain of a vertebrate animal is the most complex structure in any living organism. The versatility and analytical abilities of that structure are suggested under the microscope by the appearance of individual neurons, or nerve cells. Each such cell appears to be different from its neighbors in its elaborate form and its links with other neurons by means of synapses at the tips of its axon, or nerve fiber. There is nonetheless a remarkable consistency imposed on this diversity. As more is learned about the patterns of connectivity in various parts of the brain, principles of organization begin to emerge, raising the hope that the types of neuronal interactions underlying the apparent complexity will turn out to be manageably small in number.

One such principle of organization is mapping. The axons that project from neurons in one region of the brain to neurons in another region generally reproduce neighborhood relations. As a result if two neurons are neighbors in the first region, their synapses will form on the same cell or on neighboring cells in the second region: the target population.

This regularity in axonal projections was initially detected in the 19th century. It has now been found in all the projections through which sensory signals reach the cerebral cortex, in the projections through which one area of the cerebral cortex is connected to another and in the projections through which the parts of the brain involved in the control of movement act on the muscles of the body.

A second principle of organization, much more recently recognized, is the partitioning of the regions of the brain that embody a map into periodic subdistricts. For example, work in the laboratory of Jon H. Kaas at Vanderbilt University has revealed a highly regular partitioning of the somatic sensory cortex: the part of the cerebral cortex that gets sensory data from muscles, joints and the skin. In the somatic sensory cortex the surface of the hand is represented by a map. Hence touching two points on the skin that are near each other elicits measurable electrical activity in groups of neurons that are neighbors in the cortex. In experiments with monkeys Kaas and his colleagues find that in the layer of the cortex where the entering axons make their synapses, designated Layer 4, the map is partitioned into bands. The bands separate sensory inputs from the hand according to the kinds of information the input carries. In some bands the neurons respond only to the onset of a touch; in the intervening bands the neurons have a more prolonged response. It is as if the map of the hand in the somatic sensory cortex of the monkey has been constructed by alternating stripes cut out of two distinct maps of the hand. One map (and one set of stripes) represents what are called rapidly adapting nerve endings in the skin; the other represents more slowly adapting nerve endings.

Edward G. Jones and his colleagues working at the Washington University School of Medicine were among the first to demonstrate anatomically that such functional subdivisions arise because each subdivision receives particular axons. Jones and his colleagues employed a radiographic technique. They injected into the somatic sensory cortex on one side of the brain of a monkey a small quantity of amino acids labeled with tritium, the radioactive isotope of hydrogen. The amino acids were taken up by neurons in the cortex and transported down the axons projecting from some of those neurons to the somatic sensory cortex on the opposite side of the brain. There the labeled axons laid down a pattern of radioactivity that was detectable by coating slices of the tissue with a photographic emulsion sensitive to radioactivity.

The pattern of radioactivity in successive slices indicated that the axons terminate in a clearly delimited series of stripes. Thus inputs crossing from one side of the brain to the other as well as inputs carrying information from the skin terminate in stripes in the somatic sensory cortex. The partitioning of inputs to the somatic sensory cortex is not, however, the only example of striped patterns. There are many other examples. Stripes have been found in all sensory pathways, in many regions of the cerebral cortex and in regions of the brain as diverse as the superior colliculus, the cerebellum and the medulla oblongata.

Periodic synaptic zones that form functional stripes in a region of the brain that simultaneously embodies a map present a puzzle. Why are they there? Why should the brain establish an elaborate means of segregating various inputs when ultimately the inputs will converge to produce a unified representation? The two of us have done a

series of experiments that suggests an answer to the question.

Our work focuses on the visual system, a set of projections that carry visual information from the retina to more central stations of the brain. These pathways have been studied intensively, and as a result more is known about the central nervous system's representation of the visual world than is known about the representation of any other sensory modality. Much of the work was done, on the cat and the monkey, by David H. Hubel, Torsten N. Wiesel and their colleagues working at the Harvard Medical School. Their results constitute a detailed analysis of the relation between topographic and functional organization. In the cat and the monkey the visual pathways convey information to the part of the cerebral cortex designated the visual cortex. The map there is binocular: it arises from axons delivering information from each of the animal's eyes. Hubel and Wiesel found, however, that when a microelectrode is passed through brain tissue in Layer 4 of the visual cortex, it records the electrical activity of neurons in a highly regular alternating sequence. An initial series of neurons might respond only to flashes of light in the animal's left eye. Then would come a series of cells responding only to the right eye, and then again a series of cells responding to the left.

Hubel, Wiesel and their colleagues further showed that this functional alternation results from the segregation of the axons that carry information from each eye. The labeling of each eye's visual pathway with radioactive amino acids reveals stripes that run in a zebralike pattern throughout Layer 4 of the visual cortex (see Figure 4.1). Each stripe contains cells that respond exclusively to one eye, the left or the right. The cells in turn project their axons to binocular neurons in the cortical layers above and below them. In other words, every part of the visual world on which the cat or the monkey can train both of its eyes is represented twice in Layer 4: once at some point in a stripe of cells representing the left eye and again in a neighboring stripe representing the right eye.

Our own experiments at Princeton University capitalized on several properties of a considerably different visual pathway, that of the leopard frog (*Rana pipiens*). The experiments relied on a classical procedure of transplanting tissue in amphibian embryos. This transplantation, however, is combined with modern techniques of neuroanatomy and neurophysiology for examining the patterns of connec-

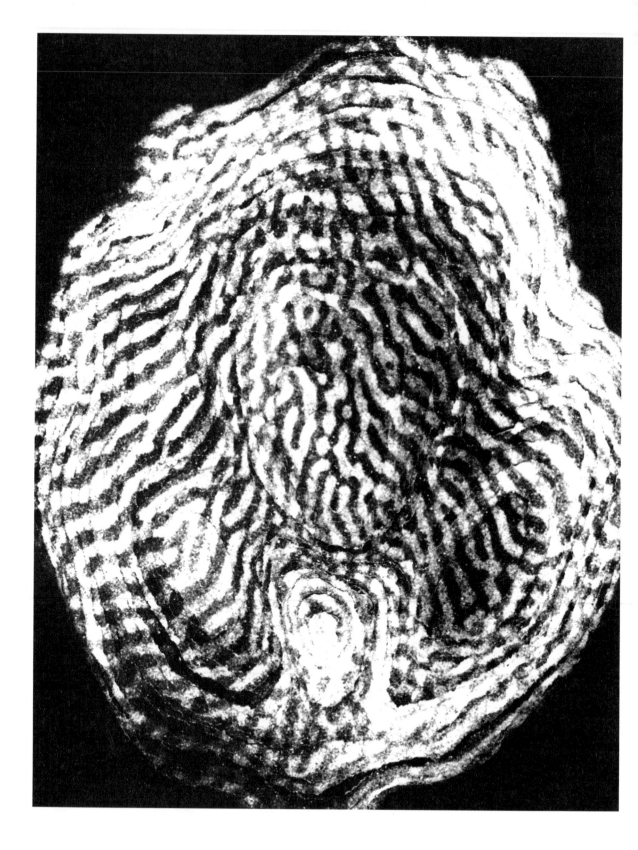

Figure 4.1 STRIPES IN A MAMMAL'S BRAIN are found in the visual cortex. The montage of successive slices of tissue shown is about a fourth of the visual cortex on one side of the brain of a macaque monkey. One of the animal's eyes has been injected with a small quantity of an amino acid (proline) labeled with tritium, the radioactive isotope of hydrogen, and over a period of two weeks the radioactivity has been carried in axons, or nerve fibers, from the eye to the lateral geniculate nucleus of the brain and from there to the visual cortex. When slices of tissue from the visual cortex are coated with a photographic emulsion, the radioactivity exposes the emulsion in bright stripes. The stripes interdigitate with darker stripes representing the uninjected eye. Each stripe is about 350 micrometers wide. The image was provided by Simon LeVay.

tions that neurons in the visual system make when they are placed in abnormal situations early in development. On occasion such analyses can reveal principles of growth and organization that are not obvious during normal development.

In one series of experiments we removed an eye primordium (the tissue that becomes an eye) from young embryos at a time when the eye was merely an outpouching of the embryonic central nervous system (see Figure 4.2). We then transplanted the primordium into a second embryo in the region of its own two primordia. The embryos we treated in this way became tadpoles and then young frogs with three quite normal eyes. The supernumerary eye usually ended up in front of one of the normal eyes. Sometimes it was at the end of the nose or on top of the head (see Figure 4.3).

Leopard frogs rely heavily on vision, but unlike cats or monkeys their brains have not evolved the elaborate visual cortex that is characteristic of mammals. Instead the major area for the processing of visual information is in the optic tecta, a symmetrical pair of lobes that occupies much of the midbrain. Each optic tectum receives almost all its retinal axons from only one eye, the contralateral one (the

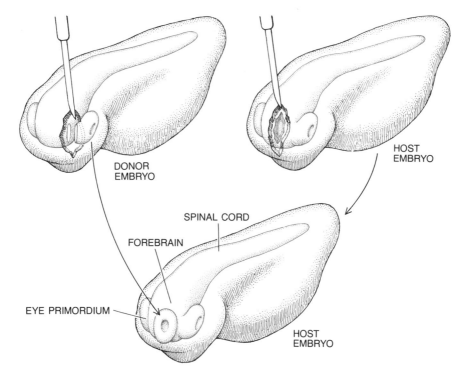

DONOR EMBRYO

HOST EMBRYO

SPINAL CORD

FOREBRAIN

EYE PRIMORDIUM

HOST EMBRYO

Figure 4.2 SURGICAL PROCEDURE that produces a three-eyed frog requires that an eye primordium be taken from one frog embryo and introduced into a second embryo after tissue has been removed to make room for it. At the time of the transplantation each embryo is some three millimeters long and each eye primordium is an outpouching from the developing forebrain.

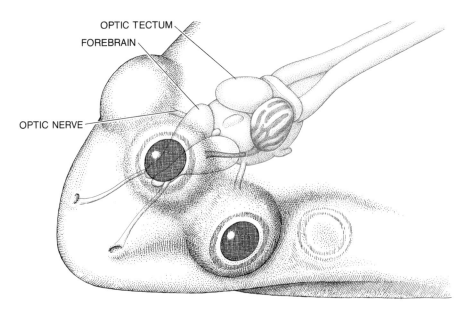

OPTIC TECTUM
FOREBRAIN
OPTIC NERVE

Figure 4.3 MATURE THREE-EYED FROG has two normal eyes positioned correctly on its head and a third eye either in front of a normal eye or on top of the head. In about three-fourths of all cases the third eye competes with a normal eye to establish axon terminals in one tectum.

eye on the opposite side of the animal's head). The projection from this eye creates a highly ordered map of the retinal surface, but since the tectum gets no massive projection from the second retina, there are no stripes representing each eye.

The three-eyed frogs are different. In most of them the retina of the supernumerary eye sends axons predominantly to one optic tectum or the other. There the supernumerary axons compete with the normal input to the tectum: the axons arriving from one of the frog's normal eyes. We examined the brain of the three-eyed frogs by injecting radioactively labeled amino acids into either the normal eye or the supernumerary one and waiting a day or two for the isotope to be transported down the axons to their synaptic terminals in the tectum. The tectal lobes of these animals were then sliced and the slices were treated to reveal the distribution of labeled synaptic terminals (see Figure 4.4).

The two sets of terminals (labeled and unlabeled) never mixed in a slice. Instead they were segregated into eye-specific zones that interdigitated periodically. Moreover, a tracing of the zones of labeled terminals through successive slices showed that the zones were aligned into stripes. Each stripe was

about 200 micrometers wide and ran roughly from the front to the back of each lobe in a zebralike pattern. The pattern was always similar. It made no difference whether the supernumerary eye came originally from the right or the left side of a donor embryo or whether the axons from the supernumerary eye grew into the right or the left optic tectum. The trajectory taken by the supernumerary axons, the way they bundled together as they grew and the direction from which they entered the tectal lobe also made no difference.

In a related experiment several laboratories as well as our own removed one of the two tectal lobes from a normal frog or a goldfish. The axons from the retina that had projected to the missing lobe regenerated. They grew into the remaining tectum, where they competed with the projection already there and produced alternating stripes of terminals arising from axons of the left and the right eye. The experimental doubling of visual input to a tectal region that usually supports only one map of the retina seems inevitably to produce in a lower vertebrate animal a set of complex functional subdivisions that are strikingly similar to the pattern in the visual cortex of normal mammals.

In some of our three-eyed frogs we recorded the

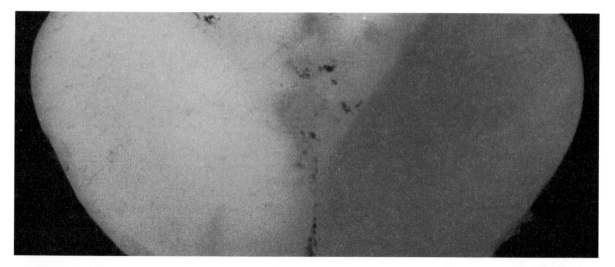

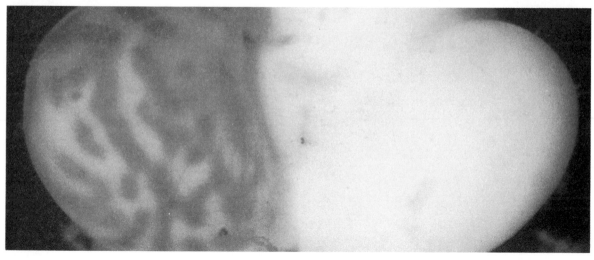

Figure 4.4 STRIPES in the brain of the leopard frog are revealed by injecting the enzyme horseradish peroxidase into one of the optic nerves so that it is transported into the brain. The brain is then treated so that the enzyme produces a brown reaction product inside the terminals of the axons. The top photo shows the optic tectums of a normal frog. The optic nerve from the left eye has been injected with the enzyme; thus the tectum on the right is marked with reaction product. The even tone of brown suggests that the axons projecting to the tectum distribute their terminals there continuously. In this way the tectal cells embody a topographic map of the retina. The bottom photo shows the brain of a frog that developed with three eyes. The supernumerary axons have been injected with the enzyme; they can be seen in the tectum, where their terminals are in stripelike regions. The stripes alternate with stripes of the terminals of axons from the normal eye. (Photo by the authors.)

activity at the terminals of retinal axons in the tectum while we flashed spots of light on a screen in front of the frog (see Figure 4.5). First we covered the normal eyes and then the supernumerary eye. In this way we could show that each eye's representation on the doubly innervated tectum was properly aligned with respect to the original axes of the eye in the embryo. Thus the axons in each projection maintained in the tectum a map of the retina from which they arose even though the map is interrupted by the interdigitating stripes (see Figure 4.6). Here again the abnormal frogs resemble the

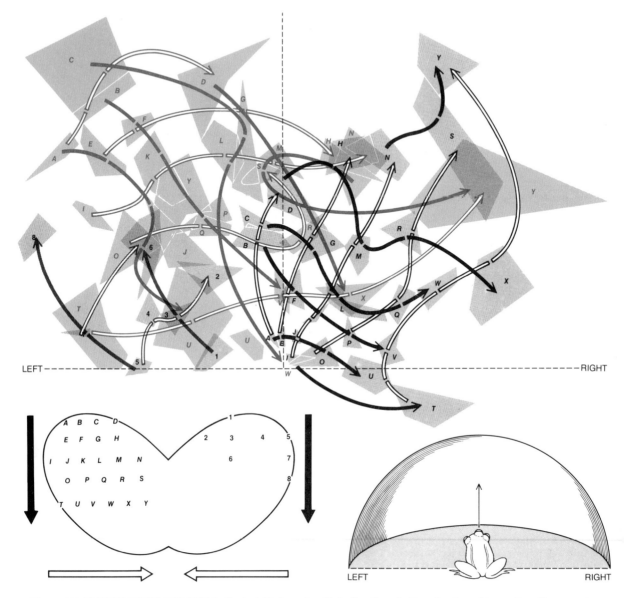

Figure 4.5 ORIENTATION OF MAPS in the tectal lobes of a three-eyed frog is determined by recording the electrical activity of groups of retinal axons as lights are flashed at various places on a hemispherical surface in front of the frog. Numbers *1* through *8* mark sites at which recordings were made in the right tectum and receptive fields. The right tectum embodies a map of the world seen through the eye on the left side of the head (*gray*). Open arrows link directions in the visual world monitored by axon terminals arrayed from side to side in the tectum; closed arrows link directions monitored by axon terminals arrayed from front to back. The letters *A* through *Y* mark sites of recording in the left tectum and the receptive fields. The left tectum embodies two maps, that of the normal right eye (*black*) and that of the supernumerary eye (*color*).

normal mammal. Two retinal inputs produce two separate representations of the visual world in a single target structure.

In a mammal, however, the two eyes are symmet-

rically positioned on the head. This is not the case in a three-eyed frog, where the supernumerary eye is positioned abnormally on the head. In a three-eyed frog the projection from the supernumerary retina to the tectum generally transmits a view of the animal's surroundings that is improperly matched to the view from the normal retina. This means that neurons near each other but in adjacent stripes in the tectum get information about unrelated parts of visual space. The situation could be simulated by fitting one of your own eyes with a prism that bent the light to that eye by, say, 90 degrees. As you looked around, the prism would transmit images from the sky above you into one eye while the other eye saw the terrain in front of you. Both images would be signaled simultaneously to the same part of the visual cortex. The world would make little sense.

A three-eyed frog presented with an erratically moving object that mimics its prey (a flying insect) often remains immobile. Occasionally it strikes aberrantly at the stimulus. If the frog is allowed to see through its normal eyes but not the supernumerary one, the strikes are accurate. Presumably the tectal maps representing the normal eyes are correctly aligned with the motor pathways in the nervous system that control the frog's behavior. If the frog is allowed to see through only the supernumerary eye, the strikes are always misdirected. The motor pathways driven by the misaligned visual map move the animal's body in directions that are inappropriate to the prey's position in space.

Questions about the functional or evolutionary significance of stripes in the brain of three-eyed frogs are clearly irrelevant. The third eye is abnormal, and in the absence of substantial input from both of the normal eyes to a single optic tectum the normal frog would get no benefit from a mechanism that evolved specifically to segregate tectal inputs into stripes. On the other hand, the survival of free-living frogs, and in particular their ability to catch the insects on which they feed, depends critically on a robust mechanism to ensure that a precise map of the contralateral retinal surface develops in each tectum (see Figure 4.6).

We began, therefore, to consider the possibility that stripes might arise from the same developmental mechanism that generates maps. Such a link was first suggested as early as 1975 by Simon LeVay, working in collaboration with Hubel and Wiesel at the Harvard Medical School. LeVay proposed that the functional stripes in the visual cortex of the monkey might represent a compromise between two conflicting tendencies: a spreading process in which the axons carrying information from each of the retinas try to fill the entire visual cortex with a map, and a grouping process in which the axons carrying information from each of the retinas try to remain together, as if they were repelled by the inputs from the other eye. The most likely result of the two conflicting tendencies would be interdigitated stripes because a striped configuration would simultaneously optimize both processes.

What, then, are the mechanisms that give rise to neural maps? How could these mechanisms give rise to stripes when two populations of axons map themselves in a single target zone? Fortunately the projections from the retina to the optic tectum of lower vertebrate animals have long been the subject of studies of neural mapping. R. W. Sperry of the California Institute of Technology was one of the first investigators. Sperry surgically rotated the eyes of newts 180 degrees. In some of the animals he left the optic nerves intact; in others he severed the optic nerves and allowed them to regenerate. In either case the newts made errors of 180 degrees when they snapped at stimuli, and the errors did not improve as time passed. The animals behaved as if they were unaware that their retinas had been rotated. Evidently each part of the retina continued to project its axons to a particular part of the tectum, in spite of the fact that Sperry had intervened so that each part of the retina now monitored abnormal parts of the visual world. Numerous later studies expanded on Sperry's work to show that the part of the tectum that will be innervated by a particular part of the retina is determined in the embryo even before the axons leave the retina and grow into the developing brain.

In 1963 Sperry proposed a theory to explain the consistent alignment of visual maps in the brain. He suggested that retinal cells and tectal cells develop in ways that depend on their position along each of two axes in the retina and the tectum respectively, so that each cell comes to have on its surface a unique set of marker molecules. Axons from the retinal cells can then synapse only with the tectal cells that bear the complementary markers. In short, Sperry visualized a rather rigid chemical-affinity matching between the retina and the tectum. The matching, however, cannot be absolute. Experiments on fishes and amphibians in several laboratories have shown that under some conditions retinal axons synapse with tectal neurons that are not their normal targets. A retina reduced to half its size by surgery can send its axons to form an expanded projection across an entire tectal lobe. Conversely, the axons from an entire retina can compress their

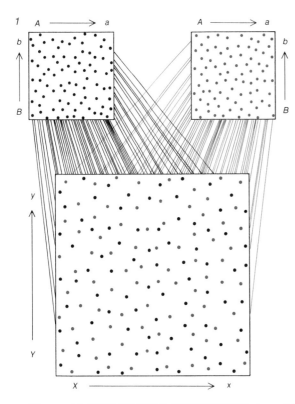
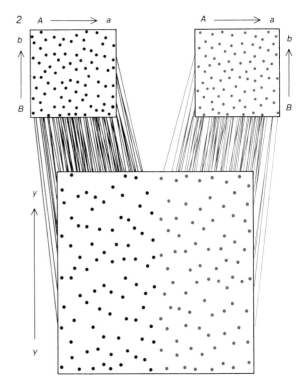

Figure 4.6 CONCEIVABLE MECHANISMS by which maps in the brain develop are compared. Two retinas are at the top of each part of the illustration. Their cells (*dots*) are assumed to be labeled by gradients in the concentration of two substances (*A, B*) on the surface of the cells. A tectum to which the retinas send their axons is at the bottom of each part of the figure. In the simplest form of the mecha-nism called chemoaffinity matching (*1*) the cells in the tectum are labeled by gradients (*X, Y*) whose complemen-tarity to the retinal markers guides the ingrowing axons. The axons from both eyes mix as they establish terminals in the tectum, a result that is never found in three-eyed frogs. In mechanism *2* the axons from each retina maintain their spatial order as they grow toward the tectum. The

map so that it will occupy a surgically created half tectum.

Clearly a mechanism based on a rigid matching of fixed markers on retinal and tectal cells cannot account for the plasticity indicated when the sizes of the retinal and tectal cell populations are surgically altered. Instead the positions of retinal axons in the tectum must be controlled by some mechanism that can adjust to changes in the relative numbers of retinal and tectal cells.

How is the adjustment accomplished? Three possibilities have been formulated. First, the rigid chemoaffinity markers proposed by Sperry could be capable of "respecification," so that surgical perturbation could cause the marker in the retina or the tectum to change. Second, instead of depending on many different markers the identification of cells in the retina or the tectum could depend on gradients of two marker substances, one along each of two axes.

The third possibility is that the retina and the tectum have no markers at all. Instead the axons projecting from the retina to the tectum might maintain their relative order by a cohesion they maintain among themselves as they grow toward the tectum. One must then explain how the map as a whole comes always to have the same orientation in the tectum. In particular the retinal maps in all nonmammalian vertebrate animals represent the central part of the animal's visual world in the anterior (forward) part of the tectal lobe and the more

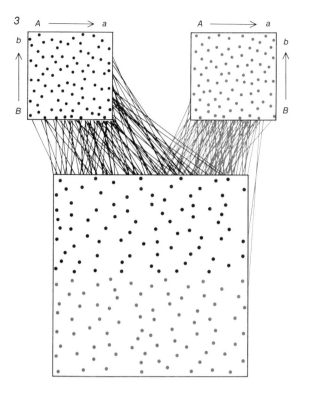

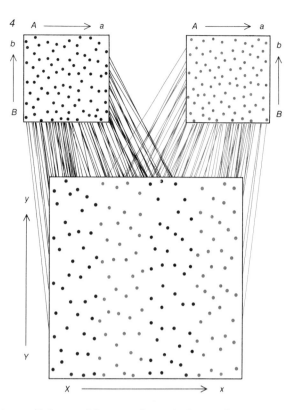

tectum itself provides only enough information (in this case a single gradient) to orient the map. Each retina innervates a separate district of the tectum, a result that is actually never found. In mechanism *3* the axons maintain their order but get no information from the tectum. In this instance they produce rotated maps. That too is never found. Two processes operate in mechanism *4*. First an imprecise

chemoaffinity matching spreads terminals over the tectum in proper orientation. Then a set of local interactions maintains as neighbors in the tectum only the terminals of axons arising from cells that are neighbors in one of the retinas. Stripes are the result because only stripes simultaneously optimize each of the two processes.

lateral parts of the visual world in the posterior parts of the lobe.

Several lines of evidence are now available to help in evaluating these various possibilities. Indeed, the first possibility, the idea of changing or respecifying rigid retinal or tectal markers, may not be apt. For one thing a series of surgical manipulations done on goldfish in a number of laboratories has shown that a tectum can sequentially receive input from a normal retina, then from an expanded half retina, then from a normal retina again. In addition there are a few reports of experiments on frogs of the genus *Xenopus* in which a region of tectum (although possibly not the same tectal cells) simultaneously receives input from the embryonically anterior half of one retina and the embryonic-

ally posterior half of the other retina. Thus if tectal labels respecify, they are capable of doing so frequently. Moreover, the cells within a small region of the tectum can change their labels independently of their neighbors. The tectal markers must be so plastic that they could not identify a cell by its tectal position.

For their part, the markers in the retina, if they exist at all, do not seem to change. Scott E. Fraser, working at Johns Hopkins University, removed an eye from tadpoles of the frog *Xenopus*. The intact eye then projected axons to the contralateral tectum just as it would have done normally. In addition the ventral (lower) part of the intact eye, whose contribution to the optic nerve was still developing at the time of the surgery, sent axons to the full extent of the ipsilateral tectum, the one that would have been innervated by the eye that had been removed. If a ventral region of a retina can project an expanded map to one tectum and a normal map to the other, it must connect to cells in different tectal positions. This makes it unlikely that the expansion of a map involves the respecification of retinal markers.

The second possibility, that of graded markers in the retina and the tectum, accounts for expansions or compressions of a map. It accounts for the ability of cells in a given region of the tectum to receive axons from different parts of a retina. It also accounts for the ease with which a part of a retina can send axons to quite different parts of two tectal lobes. A separate gradient of a marker molecule along each of two axes is sufficient to provide each retinal and tectal position with a unique combination of markers, and the match between retinal and tectal positions is able to adjust to the range of the markers present in the retina or the tectum.

The hypothesis of graded markers predicts, however, that the orientation of a retina's projection on the tectum is maintained after any perturbation. A few experiments show otherwise. Ronald L. Meyer, working at the California Institute of Technology, removed half of a goldfish's retina. The removal eliminated the input to half of one tectal lobe. At the same time Meyer forced half of the axons from the other eye to grow into the half-vacant tectum. One might predict that the rerouted axons would end in the half-vacant tectum much as they would end in the tectum to which they normally project. In this experiment the axons Meyer rerouted would have ended in the part of the half-vacant tectum that retained its retinal input. Instead the rerouted axons formed a misoriented (in fact inverted) projection in the vacant half of the lobe. Apparently the rerouted axons from the center of the intact eye got as close to their appropriate tectal position as possible. The other rerouted axons, however, could not preserve both the continuity and the orientation of their retinal map because that would have forced them to terminate in the occupied part of the tectum. Meyer's study indicates that preserving neighborhood relations must be an important tendency that can operate independently in forming a map. After all, in Meyer's experiment neighborhood relations were maintained in an inappropriate region of tectum and at the expense of the normal orientation of the map.

Results of this kind seem to support the third possibility, which favors a cohesion among the axons growing toward the tectum and proposes that there is no chemoaffinity matching between retinal axons and tectal cells. Proponents of the idea cite studies indicating that in fishes, frogs and chickens axons from many (but not all) parts of the retina grow toward the tectum together with axons from cells that are their neighbors in the retina. As we have noted, however, the idea does not explain why normal maps are consistently oriented. The absence of retinal and tectal markers is also difficult to reconcile with a large number of experiments in which retinal axons disrupt the continuity of their map to terminate appropriately in a piece of tectal tissue that is rotated or transplanted to an abnormal position in the tectum.

What most convinced us that retinal and tectal markers must exist was a finding we made in three-eyed frogs. In about a fourth of the frogs the supernumerary retina sent axons to both sides of the brain, so that neither tectum was completely striped. In such frogs a hole in the banding pattern in one tectum turned out to correspond to a patch of bands at the mirror-symmetrical location in the other tectum (see Figure 4.7). If ingrowing axons from a third eye simply preserve the topology of the retina, the projections to the tecta should have expanded and formed stripes throughout both lobes. Apparently, however, the supernumerary axons can compete with the axons from the normal retina for tectal space only at locations that are appropriate for the part of the retina in which the axons arise. It seems, therefore, that tectal cells are marked and that retinal axons can discriminate between the tectal labels.

Moreover, recent work in our laboratory shows that a tectum never innervated by a retina can nonetheless develop a map. We removed both eye primordia from frog embryos well before they had begun to send axons into the brain. Later we traced the axonal projections by which the tecta had established maps in other parts of the brain. The maps were identical in eyeless and normal frogs. Thus tectal cells are able to express their positional identities independently of their connections with the retina. Clearly some form of information must be available in the tectum to ensure the proper registration of the retinal map with other visual maps in the brain.

It now seems plain that no one simple mapping mechanism will resolve the controversies that emerge from the many experimental observations.

RIGHT TECTUM

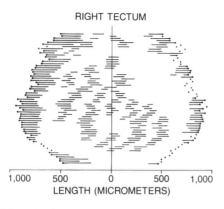

LEFT TECTUM

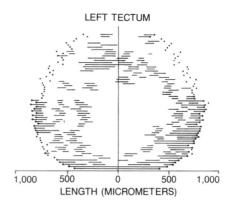

LENGTH (MICROMETERS)

Figure 4.7 MIRROR-SYMMETRICAL PATTERNS of stripes are found in a three-eyed frog in which the supernumerary eye sent axons to both optic tecta. Specifically, a hole in the pattern of stripes in one tectum corresponds to a mirror-symmetrical patch of stripes in the other. The patterns suggest that axons from the supernumerary eye compete in the tectum with axons form a normal eye only at particular parts of the tectum determined by where the axons arise in the retina. The surface of each tectum was reconstructed in the figure by measuring the widths of the stripes in a series of sections of the tectum made at intervals of 20 micrometers.

On the one hand it appears that the axons from a certain part of the eye are able to seek out a certain part of the tectum. On the other hand a number of studies (and indeed the stripes in the doubly innervated optic tectum of three-eyed frogs) reflect a cohesiveness among the synaptic terminals representing one retina that cannot be explained by any chemoaffinity matching of retina to tectum.

If one assumes, however, that two independent mechanisms operate in the establishment of neural maps, many of the controversies disappear. Moreover, striping becomes a logical extension of mapping. Suppose that early in the development of a map chemoaffinities graded along at least two axes of the retina and the tectum guide ingrowing axons. The guidance need not be precise: the gradients could be shallow and the affinities could be quite weak. In the visual system of the leopard frog one need only assume that each axon arrives in the appropriate quadrant of the tectum. The precision of the map would result from a second stage of development, in which interactions in the tectum would maintain as neighbors only those axon terminals arising from cells that are neighbors in the retina. The result of this sequence will be the compromise recognized by LeVay, Hubel and Wiesel, in which the target zone of two projections is divided into elongated terminal bands.

The appeal of chemoaffinity as a hypothesis has inspired investigators to search for marker molecules on the surface of cells in the retina and the tectum. The molecules must be distributed across the retina or the tectum with a gradient and with an ability to bind other substances that could give rise to the known alignment of the tectal map. Several recent advances promise success. For example, workers in the laboratory of Marshall W. Nirenberg at the National Heart, Lung, and Blood Institute expose cells of the immune system of the mouse to extracts of the retina of the chick. The cells in the mouse's spleen that make antibodies are then isolated and cloned. Each resulting cell culture manufactures a highly specific antibody, and one of the antibodies obtained in this way turns out to bind in a graded manner to cells along one axis of the retina. It follows that the unknown molecule to which the antibody is binding has a similar graded distribution. Taking a different experimental approach, Willi Halfter, Michael Claviez and Uli Schwartz, working at the Max Planck Institute for Viral Research in Tübingen, have addressed the question of adhesion between the retina and the tectum. They find that axons from different parts of the chick retina show consistent differences in their ability to bind membranes isolated from chick tectal cells.

Basic questions continue, however, to surround the second stage of mapping: the interactions that keep the terminals from neighboring cells together and presumably give rise to stripes. Michael P. Stryker of the University of California School of Medicine in San Francisco has shown that tetrodotoxin, a drug that blocks the ability of neurons to signal one another by means of the voltage spikes called action potentials, prevents or delays the development of stripes in the visual cortex if it is injected into the eyes of a kitten. The projections of the eyes remain mixed in their cortical target zone. N. V. Swindale of the University of Cambridge has reported similar results after raising kittens in the dark.

Apparently neural activity is essential for the cohesiveness among the synaptic terminals that represent one eye or the other. How might this work? Within a given retina neighboring cells that project their axons to the tectum (or toward the visual cortex) tend to generate similar sequences of action potentials because they are connected (by way of intermediate retinal neurons) to many of the same light-receptor cells (see Figure 4.8). Moreover, the correlated action potentials from neurons that are neighbors in the retina are more likely than uncorrelated signals to induce electrical activity in a given tectal cell. Hence well-correlated activity at pairs of synapses could conceivably serve in the tectum (or the visual cortex) to label the synapses from cells that are retinal neighbors. If the tectal neurons were

to reinforce synapses from several well-correlated neurons at the expense of synapses whose signaling is relatively ineffective, a roughly topographic map would become precise.

In sum, a two-mechanism model of how the tectal map develops proposes the existence of weak graded affinities that roughly align the retinal axons in the tectum. The map is then precisely ordered by the strengthening of synapses from neighboring retinal cells, which tend to be active simultaneously. Cristoph von der Maslberg and David Willshaw, working at the Max Planck Institute for Biophysical Chemistry in Göttingen, have devised computer simulations in which the selective reinforcement of synapses acts on two roughly topographic projections in a single target zone. They find that the simulations give rise to maps with stripes.

The idea that the efficacy of synaptic terminals can determine their stability and their position in the brain is neither recent nor limited to maps. In the 1940's D. O. Hebb of McGill University suggested that the selective strengthening of synapses might underlie certain aspects of learning. Variants of Hebb's suggestion have since been made to ac-

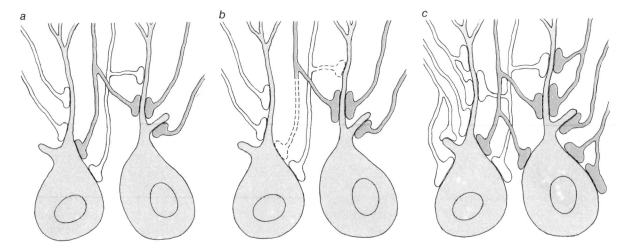

Figure 4.8 CELLULAR EVENTS thought to underlie the development of a precise tectal map are diagrammed for two cells in a tectum innervated by two eyes. An initial episode of chemoaffinity matching leaves local overlaps in which axons from different eyes impinge on the same tectal cells (a). Then the terminals representing one eye are strengthened (in the drawing they are assumed to get bigger) at the expense of terminals representing the other eye (b). In addition the density of "correct" terminals could increase (c). In either case each retina comes to dominate groups of cells. The terminals representing cells that are neighbors in a retina are likely to transmit well-correlated signals. This correlation could underlie the strengthening of precisely mapped connections and at the same time be responsible for stripes.

count for the development of neural circuitry in the cerebellum, for the sensitivity of sensory neurons to particular stimuli and for the maturation of the motor connections between the nervous system and the muscles. Although neuroscientists are still far from unraveling the molecular mechanisms that would underlie the selective strengthening or stabi-

lization of synapses, the concept itself is helpful in the effort to understand how neural activity can influence neural structure. Action potentials and the relative effectiveness of synaptic signals are quite likely to be the link between maps and stripes in the brain. They may indeed fine-tune the developing nervous system.

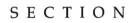

SECTION

III

EMOTION AND MEMORY

. . .

The Reward System of the Brain

Two decades ago it was discovered that the brain has "pleasure centers." These centers are now seen as belonging to a system of pathways that appear to play a role in learning and memory.

. . .

Aryeh Routtenberg
November, 1978

Neuroscientists have learned much about the anatomy, physiology and chemistry of the brain. Does this knowledge relate to human learning, pleasure and mood? Is it possible that these complex processes are mediated by specific brain pathways and specific chemical substances? The answer appears to be yes, largely as a result of an intriguing but puzzling discovery made some 20 years ago at McGill University by James Olds and Peter Milner. They demonstrated that a rat with an electrode inserted into a certain area of its brain would press a treadle to stimulate itself [see "Pleasure Centers in the Brain," by James Olds; SCIENTIFIC AMERICAN, October, 1956]. Olds, a pioneer in the study of the relation between brain function and behavior, died in a swimming accident in 1976; his death was particularly tragic because he was engaged in exciting new explorations of brain physiology.

The phenomenon discovered by Olds and Milner, which is now referred to as brain reward, can be localized in particular nerve cells and their fibers. The brain-reward system is affected by drugs that interact with the substances secreted by these nerve cells. The fact that only certain nerve-fiber pathways are implicated in brain reward suggests that these pathways have a specific function. This parallels what is known of the visual system and the movement system, each of which has a specified set of component pathways.

Olds, first at the University of California at Los Angeles and then at the University of Michigan, took the initial steps toward identifying the pathways that support brain reward. He confirmed that self-stimulating behavior in laboratory animals is prompted only by the stimulation of particular brain areas and is not a general effect due simply to the electrical stimulation of brain tissue. For example, stimulation of the medial forebrain bundle, a group of nerve fibers that pass through the hypothalamus, gave rise to the highest rates of treadle-pressing in response to the lowest electric currents: shocks from electrodes in this area could produce response rates of more than 100 presses a minute. There were also areas characterized by milder effects: for example, stimulation of the septal area caused the animals to respond only about 10 times a minute.

In 1962, while working in Olds's laboratory, I became interested in these different response rates for stimulation of different brain regions and set about studying them. A rat was given a choice between two treadles, one delivering rewarding brain stimulation and the other delivering the only food available to the animal during the experiment. I found that the animals would forgo food essential to their survival in order to obtain brain stimulation. This behavior was observed, however, only if the electrode was within the medial forebrain bundle (see Figure 5.1). If the electrode was as little as half a millimeter away from this area, or in other areas whose stimulation yielded a reward, such as the septal area, the animals pressed both the food-delivering and the brain-stimulation treadles and were able to maintain their body weight and survive.

I wondered whether an animal more intelligent than the rat, if it were placed in the same situation, would show the same maladaptive behavior or whether its more highly developed cerebral cortex would enable it to achieve a balance between self-stimulation and feeding. Eliot Gardner and I were able to demonstrate self-starvation in the rhesus monkey, an animal with a cortex far more advanced than that of the rat. This powerful effect implies that higher primates, perhaps even human beings, will stop eating in order to obtain rewarding brain stimulation. Such results suggest that the neural mechanisms subserving self-stimulation exert a powerful and perhaps dominant influence on behavior, particularly activities of the moment. Since the behavior is so compulsive, one wonders whether the reward system may play a role in drug addiction. For example, there is some evidence that certain regions of the brain that are sensitive to morphine and contain the morphinelike substance enkephalin are in the same location as the regions supporting brain reward.

The brain's functioning is obscured by its enormously complex array of nerve cells and their fibers, and so in order to identify the cells involved in self-stimulation it is necessary to combine the study of brain reward with the study of brain anatomy. In my laboratory at Northwestern University we have been pursuing this approach by making lesions with the stimulating electrode under light anesthesia at brain sites in rats where self-stimulation has been demonstrated. Within a few days the neural elements near the tip of the stimulating electrode begin to degenerate. We then perfuse the animals with formaldehyde, use a special stain for degenerating tissue and see which neural elements are associated with the reward effects.

An example of this approach linking self-stimulation to specific pathways is provided by our study of the cerebral cortex in the frontal lobe of the brain. Although it had been doubted that the frontal cortex was important to brain reward, there are two regions of it in the rat that we have found to support self-stimulation. We made lesions at frontal-cortex self-stimulation sites and traced a pathway through the caudate nucleus and the internal capsule on its medial side. At the level of the hypothalamus this pathway is intermingled with the medial forebrain bundle. This work offers evidence that brain reward in the medial forebrain bundle results from stimulation of these frontal-cortex fibers. There is reason to believe from other work that this system may be only one of several brain-reward systems passing through the medial forebrain bundle.

The involvement of the frontal cortex in brain reward has been demonstrated in monkeys as well as in rats. Edmund Rolls of the University of Oxford has discovered self-stimulation points in the frontal cortex of the squirrel monkey similar to the regions that have been mapped in the rat. Even though the brain locations where self-stimulation has been observed are similar in a rodent (the rat) and a primate (the squirrel monkey), the great difference among species in the size of the frontal cortex creates the potential for great variation in the significance to a given species of brain-reward stimulation.

Brain reward can be found not only in the frontal cortex and the hypothalamus but also deep within the brain stem: in the pons and the medulla. Such findings indicate that although brain reward is present only at specific locations, it extends from the forebrain to the midbrain and into the hindbrain. In 1969 Charles Malsbury and I showed that self-stimulation could be obtained with electrodes positioned in the output pathway of the cerebellum and at sites in the dorsal pontine tegmentum of the brain stem. Some of these regions were also close to newly discovered pathways that were associated with catecholamine neurotransmitters: substances that transmit the nerve impulse from one nerve cell to another. We therefore began to suspect that neurotransmitters of this type were involved in self-stimulation.

In 1971 Urban Ungerstedt of the Karolinska Institute in Stockholm described new catecholamine pathways in the forebrain, the midbrain and the hindbrain. He worked with the technique known as histofluorescence, in which the location of specific substances in a tissue is revealed by inducing them

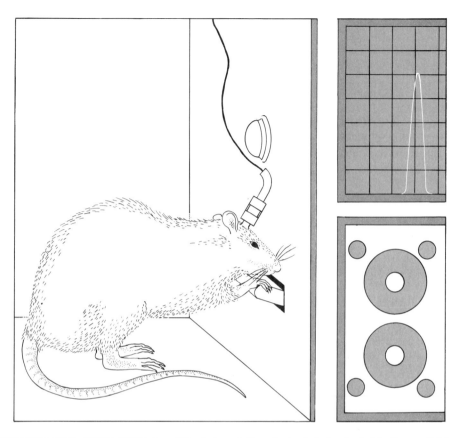

Figure 5.1 SKINNER-BOX APPARATUS is utilized to study the behavioral effects of brain reward. A metal electrode is implanted in the reward system of the rat, and the animal is allowed to trigger an electric stimulus to its brain by pressing the treadle. The curve on the oscilloscope screen indicates the delivery of the stimulus. If the stimulating electrode is implanted in the medial forebrain bundle of the hypothalamus, the rat will stimulate itself nearly continuously for days, neglecting food, water and sleep. Other parts of reward system give rise to less dramatic effects.

to emit light of a characteristic color. The technique was developed in 1962 by B. Falck and N. -Å. Hillarp, who built on earlier work by O. Eränkö of the University of Helsinki and Arvid Carlsson of the University of Göteborg. In 1974 Olle Lindvall and Anders Björklund of the University of Lund applied more sensitive techniques to establish the existence in the central nervous system of mammals of several pathways associated with the catecholamine norepinephrine and several pathways associated with another catecholamine, dopamine.

To obtain histofluorescent micrographs of brain tissue the tissue is first treated with aldehyde or glyoxylic acid, which react with catecholamines to form fluorophores, substances that fluoresce when they are excited by ultraviolet radiation. When a thin section of the tissue is exposed to ultraviolet in the fluorescence microscope, the fluorophore is excited and emits light. With the aid of a special wavelength detector norepinephrine can be seen to emit in the green-yellow region of the spectrum and dopamine in the green region. Although the color difference is difficult to determine without a special detector, the shape of the nerve fiber containing one substance or the other is different. Thus when the fluorescent fibers are observed in a histofluorescent micrograph, they reveal the anatomical location of the chemical substance. The histofluorescence technique is therefore based on histochemical principles: it is chemical in that it reveals brain pathways through a chemical reaction with neurotransmitters and histological in that the reaction takes place in a thin section of brain tissue on a microscope slide.

The existence of catecholamine pathways has been confirmed by the application of histofluorescence to the human brain (see Figure 5.2). Working with tissue from an unviable fetus, Lars Olson, L. O. Boréus and Ake Seiger of the Karolinska Institute and Hospital have found the analogous catecholamine brain pathways in humans that have been observed in the brain of rats and monkeys.

The evidence for the similar location of catecholamine pathways and areas of self-stimulation is not the sole reason for supposing there is a connection between catecholamines and the brain-reward system. The rate at which rats with an electrode implanted in their brain will press a treadle to stimulate themselves is affected by certain drugs that are known to interfere with the function of catecholamines. The same drugs are also known to affect mood in human beings; indeed, they are sometimes administered to control anxiety and psychotic behavior. Since there is a connection between these mood-altering drugs and the catecholamines and also between the catecholamines and the brain-reward system, there would seem to be one between the brain-reward system and mood and personality.

Norepinephrine and dopamine (see Figure 5.4) are two major catecholamines that have been identified as neurotransmitters in the brain. When a nerve cell in a catecholamine system is activated, it releases one of these substances. The neurotransmitter crosses the synapse, the gap between the axon terminal of one nerve cell and the cell body of the next nerve cell. In so doing it changes the permeability of the membrane of the second nerve cell to ions in the extracellular fluid and so changes its excitability. The catecholamine is then either destroyed by an enzyme or is taken back into the axon terminal of the first cell.

Drugs that manipulate the catecholamine system have a powerful effect on mood. It is generally believed such drugs act to modify catecholamine transmission at the synapse, thereby altering the neurotransmitter's ability to influence other nerve cells. Studies involving a variety of drugs that modify catecholamine synaptic transmission have revealed a straightforward relation: agents that elevate catecholamine levels or mimic the action of catecholamines facilitiate self-stimulation; agents that lower these levels depress self-stimulation. For

Figure 5.2 TWO TYPES OF NERVE FIBERS in the frontal cortex of the human brain are revealed in these images obtained by chemically treating thin sections of brain tissue so that the neurotransmitter substances in the nerve fibers fluoresced when they were illuminated with ultraviolet radiation. The top micrograph shows a nerve fiber containing dopamine. The green-fluorescent dopamine fiber is typically thin and sinuous, with irregularly spaced spindle-shaped swellings. (The bright yellow blobs in the background represent granules of the fatty pigment lipofuscin.) The bottom micrograph shows a nerve fiber containing norepinephrine, which can be distinguished from the dopamine fiber by the closely spaced swellings, which are intensely fluorescent. Micrographs are magnified approximately 900 diameters and were made by Brigitte Berger.

example, the drug d-amphetamine potentiates both the action of catecholamines and self-stimulation. The drug chlorpromazine blocks the action of catecholamines and also blocks self-stimulation.

Chlorpromazine has been effective as an antipsychotic agent, and so a link has been suggested between psychoses and the catecholamine-connected self-stimulation pathways. It seems possible that because of either genetic or environmental factors abnormalities in the brain-reward pathways could lead to permanent changes in mental state. Larry Stein and C. David Wise, working at the Wyeth Laboratories, have suggested that the cause of schizophrenia is an enzymatic deficiency that allows the production of a toxic substance, 6-hydroxydopamine, which destroys norepinephrine pathways thought to be associated with brain reward. They argue that these pathways, which can be seen in histofluorescent micrographs, are essential for adaptive behavioral responses. In support of their hypothesis they have demonstrated that synthetic 6-hydroxydopamine injected directly into the brain of a rat reduces the rate at which the rat presses a treadle to get a brain reward. This hypothesis is of special value because it explicitly relates schizophrenia to abnormalities in particular brain-reward pathways that contain a particular transmitter substance.

A question that has generated much interest among investigators of brain reward has to do with possible differences among the roles played by different catecholamines. Various hypotheses have been put forward: that self-stimulation is mediated solely by either norepinephrine or dopamine, that they are both involved but independently, or that

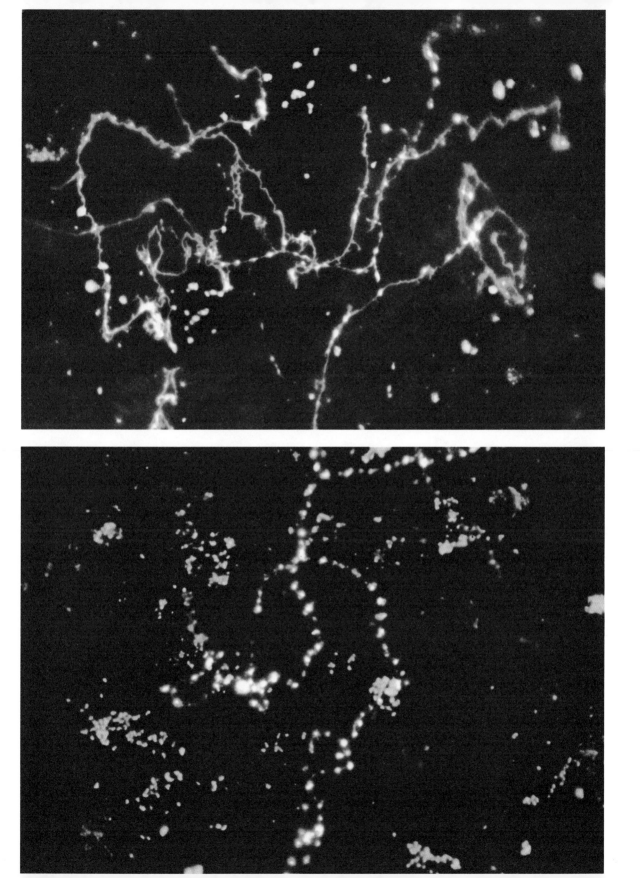

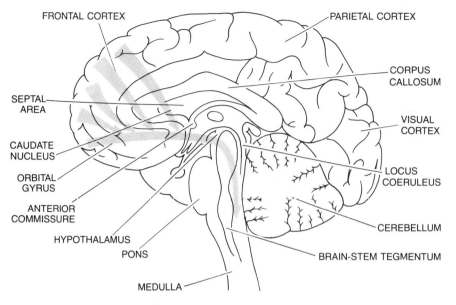

Figure 5.3 REWARD SYSTEM OF THE HUMAN BRAIN has been roughly localized in the regions shown in color. These areas correspond to the parts of the rat brain that support self-stimulation behavior. As in rodent brain, the pathways extend between hindbrain and frontal cortex.

they act in concert. Ronald M. Clavier and I have approached the problem anatomically (see Figure 5.5). We examined the contribution made to self-stimulation by two major norepinephrine systems known as the dorsal and ventral bundles. First we demonstrated that self-stimulation in the brain stem is associated with the dorsal norepinephrine bundle. We made lesions at sites that supported self-stimulation and found they gave rise to a change in the histochemical fluorescence of the dorsal bundle, indicating that this region is associated with pathways that mediate brain reward. Similar changes in the histochemical fluorescence of the ventral bundle resulted only from lesions in brain areas that were not involved in self-stimulation. Therefore whereas the ventral bundle is not associated with brain reward, the dorsal norepinephrine bundle does appear to be associated with it.

Even though the dorsal bundle is associated with self-stimulation, is it an essential component of the brain-reward system? If brain reward results from an activation of the axons in the dorsal bundle, one would expect that the destruction of the nerve-cell bodies of these axons, which are found in an area called the locus coeruleus, would reduce self-stimulation. Clavier and I found this did not happen: the

almost total destruction of the locus coeruleus had little effect on the rate of self-stimulation in rats. Interestingly enough, however, a lesion limited to the medial forebrain bundle drastically reduced self-stimulation. This effect may be related to the medial forebrain bundle's acting as a "pleasure relay station" for other brain pathways that do not contain norepinephrine.

These results indicate the norepinephrine pathways may not be critical to self-stimulation. That a dopamine system plays a more crucial role is suggested by the fact that the lesion in the medial forebrain bundle reducing self-stimulation also damaged two components of the dopamine system in the midbrain: the ventral tegmentum and the substantia nigra, pars compacta. Olds and Ephraim Peretz had shown in 1960 that the ventral tegmentum could support self-stimulation, and Malsbury and I, surveying the midbrain, the pons and the anterior medulla, had demonstrated in 1969 that the highest rates of self-stimulation were obtained from electrodes placed in the ventral tegmentum.

We also discovered brain reward in the other component of the dopamine system, the substantia nigra, pars compacta. Yung H. Huang, who was then a graduate student in my laboratory, demon-

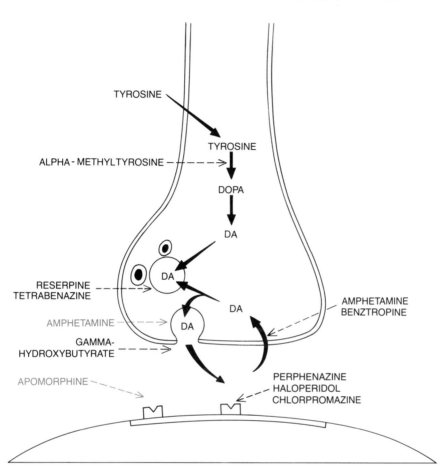

Figure 5.4 DOPAMINE TRANSMISSION across the synapse can be enhanced or inhibited by psychoactive drugs. Thus the effects of these drugs on self-stimulation behavior shed some light on the neurochemical mechanisms underlying brain reward. Dopamine transmission can be inhibited (*shown in black*) by agents that block its synthesis (alpha-methyltyrosine), prevent its storage in vesicles (reserpine, tetrabenazine), prevent its release (gamma-hydroxybutyrate) or block its attachment to receptor sites (perphenazine, haloperidol, chlorpromazine). Dopamine transmission is enhanced (*color*) by drugs that increase its release (amphetamine, cocaine), facilitate receptor activation (apomorphine) or inhibit reuptake of dopamine into the terminal from the synapse (amphetamine, benztropine).

strated the involvement of the substantia nigra by means of low currents delivered through electrode wires that were considerably smaller than those implanted in earlier experiments. C. L. E. Broekkamp of the University of Nijmegen has shown that self-stimulation in the substantia nigra is blocked by the injection into the caudate nucleus of the drug haloperidol, which selectively blocks dopamine transmission. Self-stimulation is increased by the injection of amphetamine, which enhances dopamine transmission. These results indicate that the drugs influence brain reward by acting on nerve cells in the caudate nucleus. They also indicate an important role for dopamine systems in self-stimulation mechanisms.

It has been learned only recently that both norepinephrine and dopamine systems send their axons into the cerebral cortex. This finding is a critically important one because it relates the cerebral cortex to primitive structures deep within the midbrain and hindbrain that arose much earlier in the evolu-

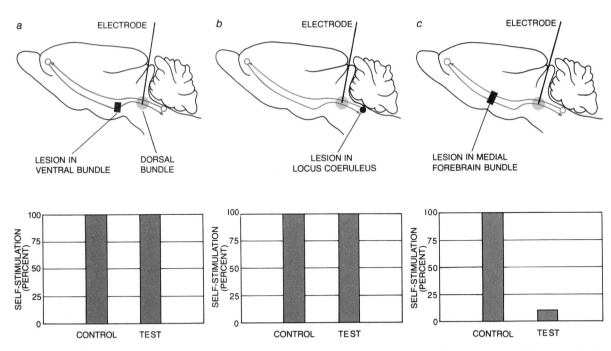

Figure 5.5 EFFECTS OF BRAIN LESIONS on self-stimulation behavior in the rat were determined in experiments performed by the author and Ronald M. Clavier. An electrode was implanted in the dorsal brain stem of the rat, and the animal was allowed to stimulate itself by pressing a treadle in a Skinner box. Lesions in the ventral bundle of the norepinephrine system (a) had no effect on self-stimulation behavior 10 days after surgery, nor did removal of the locus coeruleus (b), where the norepinephrine cell bodies giving rise to the dorsal bundle are concentrated. On the other hand, destruction of the medial forebrain bundle (c) resulted in a dramatic decline in self-stimulation, suggesting that the dopamine fibers in this region are essential for brain reward.

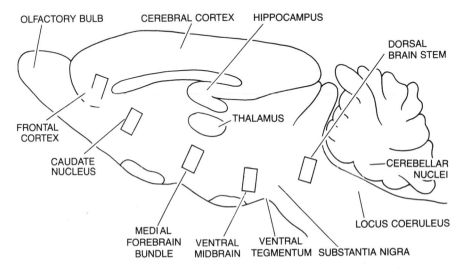

Figure 5.6 PATHWAYS OF REWARD in the rat brain are outlined schematically in this longitudinal section. The pathways extend in both directions from nerve-cell bodies in the hindbrain, the midbrain and the frontal cortex, passing through the medial forebrain bundle in the hypothalamus. The circles indicate the locations of the cell bodies; the rectangles indicate regions where reliable self-stimulation behavior has been obtained in studies with the Skinner-box apparatus.

tion of the brain. It raises the possibility that the highly complex and intricate patterns of intellectual activity in the cortex are influenced by evolutionarily primitive catecholamine systems.

By exploiting recent improvements in the sensitivity of the fluorescence technique it is now possible to distinguish between norepinephrine axons and dopamine axons in the cerebral cortex of both experimental animals and man (see Figure 5.7). There are differences in the visual appearance of the two networks: the norepinephrine fibers are thicker

and have more swellings than the dopamine fibers, which are thin and sinuous.

Although both catecholamine systems are found at self-stimulation sites, the norepinephrine system is distributed evenly throughout the layers of the frontal cortex and is found in areas where self-stimulation cannot be demonstrated. The dopamine system, on the other hand, has been shown by Brigitte Berger, Ann-Marie Thierry and Jacques Glowinski of the Collège de France to be unevenly distributed, with its highest concentration of axons and axon

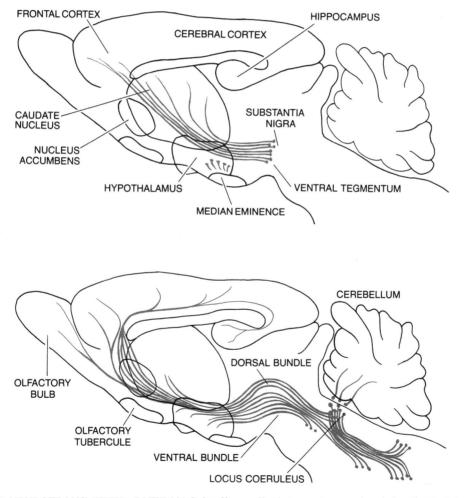

Figure 5.7 NEUROTRANSMITTER PATHWAYS implicated in the reward system of the rat brain were mapped by fluorescence microscopy. The nerve cells that secrete dopamine (*top*) have their cell bodies concentrated in the substantia nigra and the ventral tegmentum of the midbrain; their axons project primarily to the caudate nucleus, the frontal cortex and the entorhinal cortex. The nerve cells that secrete norepinephrine (*bottom*) have their cell bodies localized primarily in the locus coeruleus of the brain stem; they project to the cerebellum, the cerebral cortex and the hypothalamus. The dopamine fibers are found only in areas that mediate brain reward, whereas the norepinephrine fibers extend into other regions.

terminals located in the medial and sulcal cortex: precisely those areas in the frontal cortex where brain reward was observed. Recently Timothy Collier and I have studied islands of dopamine fluorescence in the entorhinal cortex, a region of the temporal lobe where we have demonstrated brain-reward effects.

The involvement of certain regions of the cerebral cortex in self-stimulation may therefore be related, at least in part, to their input from dopamine systems. It is tempting to think that dopamine-affecting drugs that manipulate mood and alleviate psychotic behavior may achieve part of their effect through those catecholamine systems of the cortex that support brain reward.

The fact that our recent brain-reward studies have implicated the entorhinal cortex as an area supporting self-stimulation is one of considerable interest. Fibers in this region project to the hippocampus, a brain structure thought to be involved in the formation of memory and recently shown to be connected with memory of spatial relations. A connection between brain reward and learning has been recognized since 1961, when Olds and his wife, Marianne E. Olds, showed that the stimulation of reward sites disrupted learning in experimental animals. Since then neuroscientists have gained in their understanding not only of the link between reward and learning but also of the role played by the self-stimulation pathways in memory formation.

I have speculated that the pathways of brain reward may function as the pathways of memory consolidation. By this I mean that when something is learned, activity in the brain-reward pathways facilitates the formation of memory. If these pathways are electrically stimulated in the course of the learning process, in effect jamming the circuits and altering the normal physiological activity associated with the process, one would expect memory of what is being learned to be impaired. This expectation has been confirmed to a remarkable degree by work I have done with Elaine Bresnahan, Nancy Holzman and Rebecca Santos-Anderson. We found that continuous stimulation of brain-reward regions in the medial forebrain bundle, the substantia nigra or the frontal cortex applied in the course of learning a simple task disrupts the ability of an experimental animal to remember the task 24 hours later. On the other hand, stimulation of the locus coeruleus,

which apparently is not involved in brain reward, had no effect on the retention of the task.

The involvement of the substantia nigra in memory processes is surprising because it is usually associated with the control of movement. (A malfunction of the substantia nigra has been specifically related to Parkinson's disease.) Haing-Ja Kim has shown in my laboratory, however, that injections of substances specifically overactivating the substantia nigra cause the release of dopamine and lead to the disruption of memory. It seems likely that the substantia nigra system plays a role in behavioral processes beyond the control of movement and that the system is also important in the formation of memory.

Collier and I found that the entorhinal cortex plays an interesting part in the relation between self-stimulation and memory formation. Artificial stimulation applied to this area during learning has no effect on memory, but when it is applied after learning, it impairs memory. The finding is remarkable because it means brain stimulation does not have the same effect on memory in all brain areas and at all times. The evidence from our research on the entorhinal cortex suggests that stimulation must be applied both in the appropriate brain region and at the right moment in the learning process in order to hinder memory.

One puzzling question raised by this research is that if the brain stimulation is rewarding, why does it impair learning rather than enhance it? The problem is currently being investigated, and it seems the effect is related, at least in part, to how the stimulation is administered. Norman White of McGill has shown that if animals are given the opportunity after learning to press a treadle to get rewarding brain stimulation, rather than receiving it continuously as in our memory-reward experiments, they remember the task better. The improved learning may be due to the fact that the animals self-regulate the amount of stimulation, thereby self-reinforcing their behavior. Other work also supports a view held in my laboratory, namely that this enhancement of memory is to a large extent mediated by the dopamine system of the substantia nigra.

The role of self-stimulation pathways in learning and memory remains a strong interest of several investigators of brain reward. Before his death Olds had been recording the activity of single nerve cells

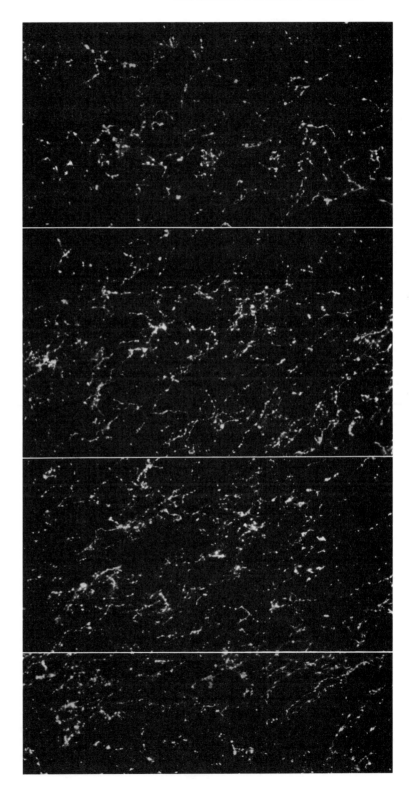

Figure 5.8 DOPAMINE FIBERS in the frontal cortex of the rat brain are revealed in this montage of fluorescent micrographs. The surface of the brain is at the top of the montage, with the deep layers at the bottom. Only dopamine fibers appear, because several weeks before the micrographs were taken a lesion was made in the locus coeruleus of the animal that destroyed all the norepinephrine fibers in the frontal cortex. Note that density of dopamine fibers is greatest in deep layers of the cortex. Micrographs were made by Olle Lindvall of the University of Lund.

DRUG	TRADE NAME	NEUROTRANSMITTERS AFFECTED	MODE OF ACTION	EFFECT ON SELF-STIMULATION	EFFECT ON LEARNING AND MEMORY
ALPHA-METHYL-TYROSINE	—	DOPAMINE NOREPINEPHRINE	INHIBITS SYNTHESIS OF CATECHOLAMINES	DECREASES RATE	IMPAIRMENT
RESERPINE	SERPASIL	DOPAMINE NOREPINEPHRINE	PREVENTS STORAGE OF CATECHOLAMINES	DECREASES RATE	IMPAIRMENT
6-HYDROXYDOPAMINE	—	DOPAMINE NOREPINEPHRINE	KILLS NERVE CELLS CONTAINING CATECHOLAMINES	DECREASES RATE	IMPAIRMENT
CHLORPROMAZINE	THORAZINE	DOPAMINE NOREPINEPHRINE	BLOCKS CATECHOLAMINE RECEPTORS	DECREASES RATE	IMPAIRMENT
AMPHETAMINE	DEXEDRINE	DOPAMINE NOREPINEPHRINE	ENHANCES RELEASE OF CATECHOLAMINES INTO SYNAPSE	INCREASES RATE	FACILITATION (AT LOW DOSES)
IMIPRAMINE	TOFRANIL	DOPAMINE NOREPINEPHRINE	PREVENTS REUPTAKE OF CATECHOLAMINES FROM SYNAPSE	INCREASES RATE	UNCERTAIN (INSUFFICIENT INFORMATION)
PHENOXYBENZAMINE	DIBENZYLINE	NOREPINEPHRINE	BLOCKS ALPHA-NOREPINEPHRINE RECEPTORS	DECREASES RATE	UNCERTAIN
PROPRANOLOL	INDERAL	NOREPINEPHRINE	BLOCKS BETA NOREPINEPHRINE RECEPTORS	DECREASES RATE	UNCERTAIN
CLONIDINE	CATAPRES	NOREPINEPHRINE	DECREASES NOREPI-NEPHRINE RELEASE	DECREASES RATE	UNCERTAIN
HALOPERIDOL	HALDOL	DOPAMINE	BLOCKS DOPAMINE RECEPTORS	DECREASES RATE	IMPAIRMENT
APOMORPHINE	—	DOPAMINE	STIMULATES DOPAMINE RECEPTORS	INCREASES RATE	FACILITATION (AT LOW DOSES)

Figure 5.9 EFFECTS OF PSYCHOACTIVE DRUGS on self-stimulation behavior and on learning and memory in the rat are summarized in this table. Drugs that enhance transmission at dopamine and norepinephrine synapses tend to potentiate self-stimulation behavior; blocking drugs tend to inhibit it. The drugs seem to have parallel effects on learning and memory, although in some cases data are inconclusive.

throughout the brain during learning in freely moving rats, and this research is being continued by Marianne Olds. James Olds had discovered certain nerve cells that "fire" 20 milliseconds or less after the presentation of a cue the animal has learned earlier is a signal for food. A number of these cells were in the substantia nigra, the region my research had connected with brain-reward pathways.

The evidence clearly shows that the brain-reward pathways play an important role in learning and memory. Much of the research strategy in the study of brain reward itself can be applied in this area, including the anatomical analysis of brain pathways and the use of drugs that affect the function of specific neurotransmitters. In this connection it is of considerable interest that certain amphetaminelike compounds potentiating the self-stimulation system are the principal therapeutic drugs prescribed for children with neurological disorders of attention and learning. These considerations suggest that as more is learned about self-stimulation pathways and their relation to learning, new therapeutic tools for assisting people with learning and memory disabilities may be discovered.

To sum up, new information about the catecholamine-fiber system has made it possible to chart the brain pathways of self-stimulation as explicitly as the pathways of well-known sensory and motor systems. Evidence for the reward effects of localized electrical stimulation, for the control of brain reward by psychoactive drugs and for the association of reward pathways with memory formation indicates that the neural substrates of self-stimulation play a vital role in the guidance of behavior. And it has been shown that reward systems are present at all levels of the brain, from the medulla oblongata to the cerebral cortex.

Since the time when the medial forebrain bundle alone was designated as the pleasure center, the boundaries of the brain-reward system have been extended deep into the brain stem and far forward into the cortex of the frontal lobe of the cerebrum. All the reward systems do, however, have pathways through the medial forebrain bundle, suggesting that this region of the hypothalamus may be described as the relay station through which the brain-reward pathways course.

It would obviously be highly desirable if brain-stimulation technology and the information derived from the study of the anatomy of the reward system could be applied to the alleviation of neurological diseases caused by disorders of the reward system. Such applications, however, have been misused in the past. All neuroscientists share the responsibility for limiting the use of brain-stimulation techniques in human beings to therapeutic purposes, and for guarding against the unwarranted or unethical applications of those techniques. Yet neuroscientists must also be prepared to communicate the positive character of their work in a society suspicious of "mind control." The potential value to society of applying such knowledge to physiological disorders of personality and mental function calls both for continued basic research and for efforts to build bridges to the clinic.

The Anatomy of Memory

An inquiry into the roots of human amnesia has shown how deep structures in the brain may interact with perceptual pathways in outer brain layers to transform sensory stimuli into memories.

. . .

Mortimer Mishkin and Tim Appenzeller
June, 1987

Within the small volume of the human brain there is a system of memory powerful enough to capture the image of a face in a single encounter, ample enough to store the experiences of a lifetime and so versatile that the memory of a scene can summon associated recollections of sights, sounds, smells, tastes, tactile sensations and emotions. How does this memory system work? Even defining memory is a struggle; introspection suggests a difference between knowing a face or a poem and knowing a skill such as typing. Moreover, the physical substrate of memory, the 100 billion or so nerve cells in the brain and their matted interconnections, is fantastically intricate. But in a tentative and schematic way, my colleagues and I (Mishkin) can begin to describe how the brain remembers.

The picture we have arrived at is largely anatomical. Over the past 20 years we have identified neural structures and stations (large arrays of cells) that contribute to memory, traced their connections and tried to determine how they interact as a memory is stored, retrieved or linked with other experience. Other investigators analyze memory on a finer scale: in some of the simplest animals and in neural tissue isolated from higher animals they have detected changes in the electrical and chemical properties of single neurons as a result of simple kinds of learning. The complexity of our subject, memory in the human brain or—as a best approximation—the brain of Old World monkeys, calls for a different initial approach, one emphasizing broad-scale architecture. Ultimately, to be sure, memory is a series of molecular events. What we chart is the territory within which those events take place.

Many of the studies leading to the current picture were suggested by case histories of patients who, because of disease, injury or surgery affecting specific areas of the brain, lost some of their ability to learn or remember. Probably the most famous of these cases is a profoundly amnesic patient known as H. M. As the subject of studies by Brenda Milner of the Montreal Neurological Institute and her colleagues from other institutions, H. M. has provided an abundance of information about the pattern of impairment associated with a specific kind of brain damage.

The experimental work, done mostly in macaque monkeys, has combined anatomical, physiological and behavioral investigations. Tracers that are carried along axons, the slender processes through which neurons send signals, have revealed the neural circuitry that might enable specific structures to play a role in memory. Measurements of the electrical activity of neurons or their uptake of radioactive glucose have distinguished parts of the brain that are active during tasks related to learning. The final category of experiment, meant to assess the functional importance of structures identified by other means, has combined surgery or drug administration with psychological testing. In the brain of an experimental animal, stations are destroyed or blocked by drugs, or the pathways linking them are severed. The animal is then examined on behavioral tests meant to tease apart the various components of memory and determine which of them is impaired.

Our route to understanding human memory is an indirect one, with unavoidable drawbacks. The macaque brain is about one-fourth the size of the brain of the chimpanzee, the nearest relative of human beings, and the chimpanzee brain in turn is only about one-fourth the size of the human brain. With the increase in size has come greater complexity. The structures we study in the macaque all have counterparts in the human brain (see Figure 6.1), but their functions may well have diverged in the course of evolution. The unique human capacity for language, in particular, and the cerebral specializations it has brought set limits to the comparative approach. Yet basic neural systems are likely to be common to monkeys and human beings, and our findings have been consistent with what is known directly about human memory loss.

THE VISUAL SYSTEM

Most often memories originate as sensory impressions. Before one asks how the brain stores a sensory experience as a memory, one would like to know how the brain processes sensory information to begin with. A study of the neural pathway responsible for visual perception was in fact the starting point for our inquiry into memory.

The central visual system begins at the striate cortex, or primary visual cortex, an area on the back surface of the brain that receives information about the visual world from the retina, by way of the optic nerve and an intermediate station (the lateral geniculate body) deep in the brain (see Figure 6.2). The striate cortex registers a systematic map of the visual field: each small region of the field activates a distinct cluster of neurons. The visual system does not end in the striate cortex, however. By the 1950's it was clear that the temporal lobe, the division of

each brain hemisphere lying behind the ear and temple, also has a role in vision.

The visual area in the temporal lobe, other workers and I learned in the 1960's, is in fact the continuation of a pathway that begins in the striate cortex. The pathway extends forward through cortical tissue (the outer layers of the brain) into the inferior temporal cortex, on the lower surface of the temporal lobe. Neuroanatomical studies showed that a number of distinct cortical stations are connected in various sequences along the pathway.

Investigators in several laboratories explored the contribution of particular stations to visual perception by surgically damaging the pathway in monkeys and then testing the animals on visual tasks, and also by recording electrical activity from each station in animals exposed to various visual stimuli. In a crucial experiment, Charles G. Gross of Princeton University and his colleagues recorded the responses of neurons in the inferior temporal cortex to stimuli—small shapes—displayed to the monkeys.

It was already known that individual neurons in the striate cortex respond most strongly to a simple stimulus, such as a short line with a specific orientation, presented at a specific location in the visual field (a phenomenon discovered by David H. Hubel and Torsten N. Wiesel). Inferior-temporal neurons recorded by Gross and his colleagues, however, responded to more complex shapes within an area averaging 20 to 30 degrees on a side. Certain neurons even responded to a complex shape wherever it was placed in the visual field. The findings suggested each inferior-temporal neuron receives data from large segments of the visual world, and often about the entire constellation of properties making up a visual stimulus.

These results and others led us to postulate that visual information is processed sequentially along the path. Neurons in the pathway have "windows" on the visual world that become progressively broader, in both their spatial extent and the complexity of the information they admit, at successive stations. The cells respond to progressively more of an object's physical properties—including its size, shape, color and texture—until, in the final stations of the inferior temporal cortex, they synthesize a complete representation of the object.

FROM EXPERIENCE TO MEMORY

Along the visual pathway, then, the brain integrates sensory data into a perceptual experience. Data

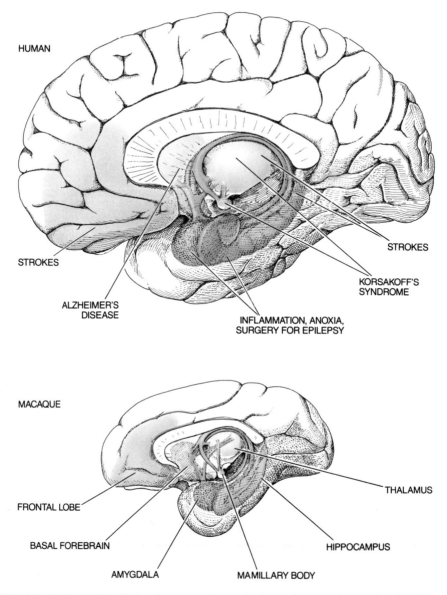

HUMAN

STROKES

STROKES

ALZHEIMER'S
DISEASE

KORSAKOFF'S
SYNDROME

INFLAMMATION, ANOXIA,
SURGERY FOR EPILEPSY

MACAQUE

FRONTAL LOBE

THALAMUS

BASAL FOREBRAIN

HIPPOCAMPUS

AMYGDALA

MAMILLARY BODY

Figure 6.1 SITES OF BRAIN DAMAGE by diseases and other events that can cause memory loss in human beings are revealed in a cutaway of the human brain (*top*). Color coding indicates the corresponding structures in a macaque brain (*bottom*), where they are labeled. The human brain is shown about two-thirds its normal size; the monkey brain is life-size.

from other senses seem to be processed in much the same way; in our laboratory at the National Institute of Mental Health, David P. Friedman, Elisabeth A. Murray, Timothy P. Pons and Richard J. Schneider recently traced an extended processing pathway for tactile sensations. At the first station individual neurons respond to single points on the surface of the body, whereas neurons in the final station respond to stimuli over broad areas and perhaps to the complete tactile experience.

What more must happen for such integrated perceptions to be stored as memory? The question is

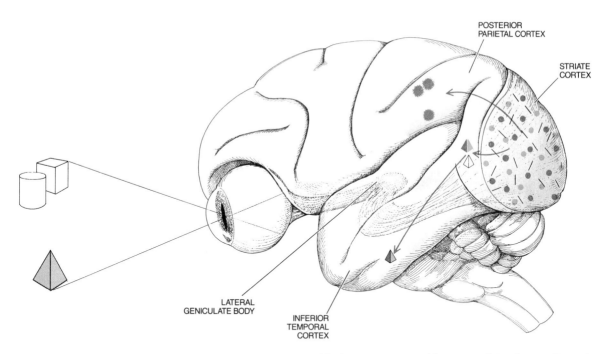

Figure 6.2 VISUAL SYSTEM processes information along two pathways, which begin in the striate cortex. Individual neurons there respond to simple, spatially limited elements in the visual field. Along the lower pathway neurons analyze broader properties of an object. At the end of this pathway, in the inferior temporal cortex, individual neurons are sensitive to a variety of properties and a broad expanse of the visual world. Along the upper cortical pathway, the spatial relations of a scene are analyzed. A perception of an object's position with respect to other landmarks would take shape in the "spatial" pathway's final station in the posterior parietal cortex.

still very much under investigation, but the crucial pathways can now be discerned. They are anchored in two structures on the inner surface of the temporal lobe in both hemispheres of the brain: the hippocampus, after the Greek word for sea horse, which the structure resembles, and the amygdala, after the Greek for almond.

Studies of human patients had already strongly suggested that the hippocampus plays a crucial role in memory. Since the 1950's the surgical removal of part of the temporal lobe has been the treatment of last resort for patients with severe epileptic seizures focused in that part of the brain. In the early days of the treatment a handful of patients developed severe amnesia after the surgery; H.M.'s handicap originated in that way. Two features of the memory loss were notable. First, the amnesia was global, extending to memory for experience in all the senses, and second, it was anterograde in nature, in that even though patients retained memories laid down some time before the surgery, they could

form no new memories. In every case of such memory loss the surgery had damaged the hippocampus.

Yet it proved impossible to reproduce a comparable, global loss of memory in animals by removing the hippocampus alone. Through a series of experiments focusing instead on the amygdala, we found that it plays as large a part in memory as the hippocampus. By damaging both structures at once, in both brain hemispheres of test monkeys, we arrived at an animal model of global anterograde amnesia.

We were motivated at first by a wish to understand just why surgical damage to the inferior temporal cortex in monkeys leaves the animals incapable of a particular kind of visual learning: choosing an object or a pattern that has consistently been associated with a reward of food over one that carries no reward. We believed the difficulty was the result of impaired visual perception, reflecting damage to the highest processing station in the visual system. Conceivably, however, the impairment instead reflected an inability to associate a stimulus with a reward.

One way to rule out the latter possibility, and thereby confirm that the difficulty of monkeys with inferior-temporal lesions was a visual one, would be to show that a different structure, undamaged in the test monkeys, is responsible for attaching reward value to a visual stimulus. With Barry Jones, then at McMaster University in Ontario, I looked for structures with which the visual system has anatomical links and tested whether surgically destroying those structures would affect the ability of monkeys to choose a baited object. Two structures we tested were the amygdala and the hippocampus, which have extensive connections (indirect ones in the case of the hippocampus) with the inferior temporal cortex.

The poor performance that resulted from bilateral removal of the amygdala suggested that it is the structure largely responsible for adding a positive association—the expectation of a food tidbit—to a stimulus processed by the visual system. Before studying the interaction of the visual system and the amygdala in greater depth, Brenda J. Spiegler, then at the University of Maryland at College Park, and I sought a way to increase the degree of impairment. We expanded the surgery to include both the amygdala and the hippocampus, whose removal by itself had had no effect.

Animals whose amygdala alone had been removed were slow to learn the association of stimulus and reward, but they were still able to do so. We were therefore startled to find that removing the amygdala and the hippocampus in combination did away altogether with the monkeys' ability to perform the task. The dramatic increase in impairment led us to wonder whether we might now be seeing a deficit that went beyond an inability to associate a familiar object with a reward. Could these monkeys have failed to choose the baited object because they could not remember the object itself from one trial to the next? That is to say, in destroying the hippocampus together with the amygdala, had we created a visual amnesia?

As it happened, Jean Delacour of the University of Paris and I had recently developed a test that was specifically sensitive to visual memory, as distinct from the ability to link an object with a reward. In that memory test, called delayed nonmatching-to-sample (see Figure 6.3), the animal is presented with a distinctive object, under which it finds a reward of a peanut or a banana pellet. Next the animal is confronted with two objects, one of them the object seen earlier and the other an unfamiliar object. The food is now concealed under the new object; the monkey is therefore rewarded for recognizing and avoiding the familiar object in favor of the novel one. Each trial makes use of a totally new pair of objects.

It is a routine that monkeys learn readily. In an adaptation of an approach developed by David Gaffan of the University of Oxford, an animal's visual memory can then be taxed by increasing the delay between the initial display and the choice or by giving the animal not one object but a series of objects to remember, followed by a series of choices. Because the food is always associated with a novel object, the ability to link a specific object to a reward has no bearing on performance. The reward serves merely as an incentive; the test measures recognition memory specifically. Normal monkeys attain almost perfect scores.

We had already applied this powerful test of visual recognition to monkeys whose inferior temporal cortex had been removed and found that the test registered the same failure to perceive or identify familiar objects that we had observed in earlier tests. We now tested animals whose visual system was intact but whose hippocampus and amygdala had been removed bilaterally. When the delay between the first object and the choice was very short, the animals could perform the task, which suggested that they suffered no defect in visual perception. When we increased the delay to a minute or two, on the other hand, their scores fell nearly to the level of chance. It seemed, then, that we had created a true memory loss.

What is more, the amnesia resulting from combined hippocampal and amygdalar lesions was not confined to visual stimuli; it seemed to be global. In our laboratory Murray found a similar impairment in the test monkeys on a nonmatching-to-sample test of tactile recognition, that is, the ability to recognize objects by touch. In human patients such global amnesia had been thought to result from damage to the hippocampus alone, and in fact a recent postmortem study of one amnesic patient by Larry R. Squire of the University of California at San Diego and his colleagues found lesions in the hippocampus only. Many other amnesic patients have more extensive lesions, however, and damage to the amygdala may have contributed to their im-

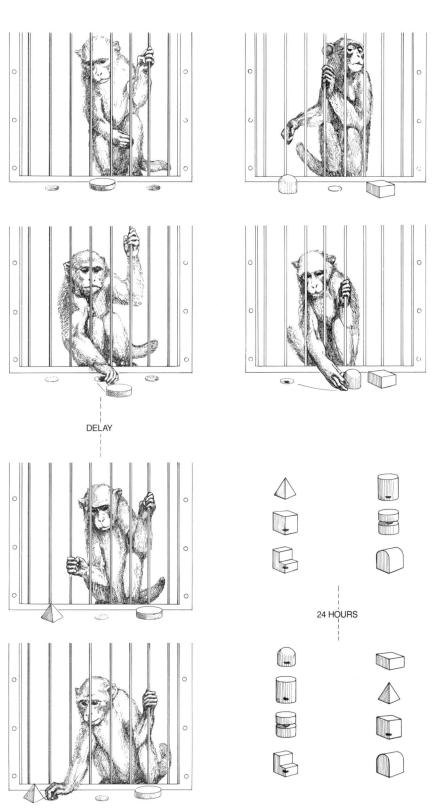

Figure 6.3 TWO TESTS OF LEARNING. In delayed non-matching-to-sample (*left*) a monkey is confronted with an unfamiliar object, which it displaces to find a reward. After a delay the animal sees the same object paired with a new one. The monkey must recognize the object it saw earlier and move the new one in order to get a reward. A second test, known as object discrimination (*right*), employs a sequence of 20 pairs of objects. One object in each pair conceals a reward. A monkey is shown the same sequence repeatedly, at 24-hour intervals, until it learns to choose the baited object in each pair consistently.

DELAY

24 HOURS

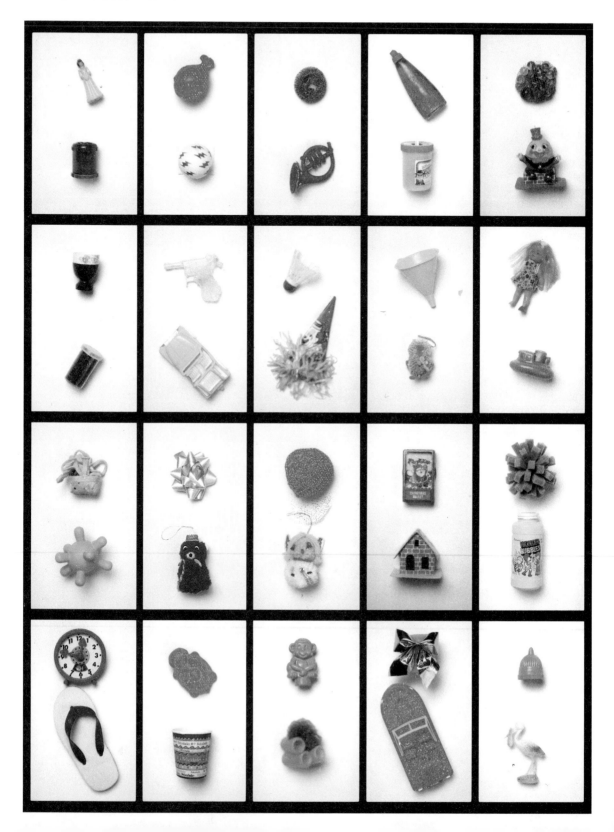

Figure 6.4 VISUALLY DISTINCTIVE OBJECTS serve for testing memory in monkeys. The author (Mishkin) and his colleagues have sought to identify the structures and pathways in the brain that enable a monkey to recognize the familiar object in a pair, having seen the object just once before. Using a plethora of objects ensures that the monkey must learn a totally new sample in each trial. (Photo by James Kilkelly.)

pairment. Indeed, an early study of amnesics suggested that the severity of their memory loss might vary in proportion to the amount of damage sustained jointly by the amygdala and hippocampus.

When we went on, with Richard C. Saunders, to examine each structure's contribution to memory in the monkey, we found just such a graded effect. In mediating visual recognition memory the amygdala and the hippocampus seem to be coequal; removing either structure by itself has only a small effect on an animal's recognition ability, presumably because each one can substitute for the other. Removing one of the structures from both hemispheres and the other from only one hemisphere yields much greater impairment. Bilateral removal of both the amygdala and the hippocampus, finally, results in an animal whose score on delayed nonmatching-to-sample is little better than chance.

FURTHER STATIONS

Damage to the amygdala and the hippocampus, two major components of what is known as the limbic system, is not the only kind of neuropathology that can result in global amnesia. In other amnesic patients the site of the damage is the diencephalon, a cluster of nuclei at the center of the brain that is organized into two structures known as the thalamus and the hypothalamus. Parts of the diencephalon situated medially (near the midline of the brain) degenerate in Korsakoff's syndrome, a global amnesia seen in some chronic alcoholics; diencephalic damage from strokes, injuries, infections and tumors can cause the same amnesic syndrome. The clinical evidence that implicates diencephalic nuclei in memory is reinforced by the anatomical finding that the diencephalon receives fibers running from the hippocampus and the amygdala.

To test the possibility that the diencephalon interacts with the limbic structures in a kind of memory circuit, we again applied our experimental stragegy of surgery followed by behavioral testing. John P. Aggleton and I destroyed, at first in combination

and then separately, the regions of the diencephalon to which the hippocampus and amygdala send fibers. Testing for visual recognition ability showed the same pattern of memory failure that had resulted when the hippocampus and amygdala were themselves removed. Combined damage to the diencephalic targets of both structures severely impaired the monkeys' recognition memory, whereas damage to either target alone had only a slight effect. It appeared we had identified two distinct memory circuits, either of which suffices for visual recognition (see Figure 6.5).

That the diencephalon and the limbic structures participate in a circuit rather than making totally independent contributions to memory was confirmed by further studies. In our laboratory Jocelyne H. Bachevalier and John K. Parkinson found that cutting the connections between the structures produced the same memory impairments seen when the structures themselves were damaged.

Earlier neuroanatomical findings suggested that we had not yet followed the circuits to their end. Nuclei in the thalamus that communicate with the limbic structures send fibers in turn to the ventromedial prefrontal cortex: an area of cortex tucked under the front of the brain. There too Bachevalier found that surgical lesions led to a profound loss of recognition memory.

Thus the final station in the visual system, and in the other sensory systems as well, is linked with two parallel memory circuits including at a minimum the limbic structures of the temporal lobe, medial parts of the diencephalon and the ventromedial prefrontal cortex. How do these structures work together in the process of memory? The question is complicated by the fact that memories are probably not stored exclusively or even mainly in the circuits themselves. The clinical observation that damage to the limbic system in humans leaves old memories intact and accessible means they must also be stored at an earlier station in the neural paths we mapped. The likeliest repositories of memory, in fact, are the same areas of cortex where sensory impressions take shape.

The subcortical memory circuits must therefore engage in a kind of feedback with the cortex. After a processed sensory stimulus activates the amygdala and hippocampus, the memory circuits must play back on the sensory area. That feedback presumably strengthens and so perhaps stores the neural representation of the sensory event that has just taken place. The neural representation itself proba-

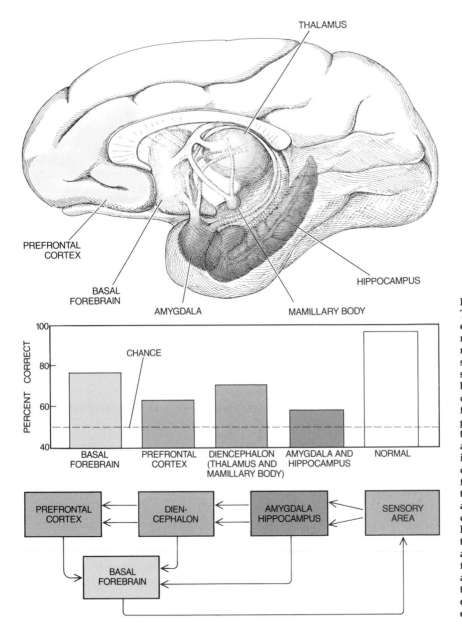

Figure 6.5 MEMORY SYSTEM was mapped largely by examining monkeys on a test measuring visual recognition memory (see Figure 6.3) after surgical damage to specific structures or pathways in the brain. The top diagram indicates structures that were found to be crucial. The graph at the middle shows the average scores monkeys achieved on the test following surgical damage to specific elements of the system; for comparison, it also shows the nearly perfect performance of normal monkeys. The chart at the bottom shows how the structures might interact in the formation of a memory. A perception formed in the final station of a cortical sensory system activates two parallel circuits, one in the amygdala and the other in the hippocampus.

bly takes the form of an assembly of many neurons, interconnected in a particular way. As a result of feedback from the memory circuits, synapses (junctions between nerve cells) in the neural assembly might undergo changes that would preserve the connectional pattern and transform the perception into a durable memory. Recognition would take

place later, when the neural assembly is reactivated by the same sensory event that formed it.

Just how each structure in the memory circuits might contribute to the feedback is not known. There are already clues to the nature of the feedback as a whole, however. One clue lies in yet another structure that our work has implicated in recognition memory. It is the basal forebrain cholinergic system, a cluster of neurons that provides the cortex and the limbic system with their major input of a neurotransmitter (a chemical messenger that carries signals across synapses) called acetylcholine.

Acetylcholine seems to play a vital role in memory. For one thing, it is depleted in Alzheimer's disease, one hallmark of which is memory loss. In our laboratory Thomas G. Aigner has found, moreover, that monkeys perform better than they normally do on the test of visual recognition memory when they are given physostigmine, a drug that enhances the action of acetylcholine. When they are given scopolamine, on the other hand, a substance that blocks the action of the neurotransmitter, their performance is impaired. Recently, in collaboration with a team of investigators headed by Donald L. Price and Mahlon R. DeLong at the Johns Hopkins University School of Medicine, Aigner and I also established that damaging the basal forebrain impairs recognition memory in monkeys, although the effect seen so far is not as severe or long-lasting as the effects of damaging the other structures we have studied.

The circuitry that would enable the other structures to enlist the basal forebrain in memory formation is certainly present. For example, the hippocampus and amygdala have extensive projections to the basal forebrain, which in turn sends acetylcholine-containing fibers back not only to the limbic structures but also to the cortex. In a plausible scenario for memory formation, the activation of the subcortical memory circuits by a sensory stimulus would trigger the release of acetylcholine from the basal forebrain into the sensory area. The acetylcholine (and probably other neurotransmitters whose release is triggered in the same way) would initiate a series of cellular steps that would modify synapses in sensory tissue, strengthening neural connections and transforming the sensory perception into a physical memory trace.

Results of a recent biochemical study suggest that a possible mechanism of synaptic modification is active in the area we believe is a likely site of memory storage: the final stations of the visual system (see Figure 6.6). Aryeh Routtenberg of Northwestern University has proposed that the addition of a phosphate group to a brain protein known as $F1$ by an enzyme, protein kinase C, underlies the synaptic changes seen after repeated electrical stimulation of certain neurons. To gauge the activity of the phosphorylation mechanism in the monkey visual system, Routtenberg and his student Robert B. Nelson added radioactive phosphorus to tissue that my group had dissected from visual areas. The largest amounts of the tracer were incorporated into $F1$ in

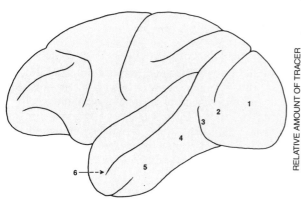
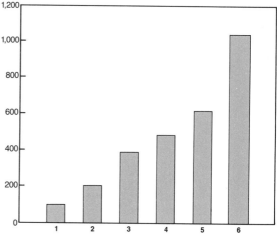

Figure 6.6 EVIDENCE OF A MOLECULAR MECHANISM that may play a role in learning reaches a peak in final stations of the monkey visual pathway. The chart, from a study led by Routtenberg, shows the relative amounts of radioactive phosphorus tracer incorporated into a protein known as $F1$ in tissue from points along the pathway. Routtenberg has proposed that phosphorylation of $F1$ by the enzyme protein kinase C underlies changes in the synapses of some neurons after repeated stimulation. Such changes may figure in data storage by the brain. Thus final visual stations may be biochemically suited to memory.

tissue from the final stations. The finding may indicate that tissue there has a special capacity to undergo synaptic changes that could store memories.

TYPES OF MEMORY

The brain architecture described so far was revealed by its contribution to one kind of memory: recognition memory, the remarkable faculty by which a monkey, having seen or felt a distinctive object just once, can recognize the object many minutes later and avoid it in favor of a novel one. There are more complex kinds of memory, of course, some of which can also be tested in monkeys. Their exploration has revealed interesting specializations in the neural paths we traced.

In perceiving an object, for example, one learns not only its distinguishing features but also its location with respect to other objects or landmarks. Remembering a sculpture seems intuitively to be a different task from remembering its position on a gallery floor. Neuroanatomically the task is different as well. To begin with, spatial vision—the ability to see spatial relations—depends on a branch of the visual system different from the one responsible for perception of an object's distinctive qualities.

In 1973, working in our laboratory, Walter Pohl confirmed earlier suggestions that tissue in the parietal cortex, near the top of the brain, has a visual role. He showed that its removal leads to a visual impairment—but a very different impairment from the one that follows damage to the inferior temporal cortex. Unlike monkeys with inferior-temporal lesions, animals with parietal damage could still tell distinctive objects apart, but they could not perceive spatial relations.

Pohl's evidence came from a test in which monkeys were presented with two covered food wells. A cylindrical object stood between the wells, closer to one well than to the other in a position that varied from trial to trial. The monkeys were rewarded for uncovering the well nearer the cylinder; it contained a peanut, whereas the other well was empty. The task is relatively easy for animals with inferior-temporal lesions. Animals with damage to the posterior parietal cortex, however, had great difficulty learning to pick the baited well.

Other work, including a metabolic study done by Kathleen A. Macko, Charlene D. Jarvis and me in collaboration with a team headed by Charles Kennedy and Louis Sokoloff, working at the National Institute of Mental Health, confirmed that the posterior parietal cortex belongs to the visual system. We injected a radioactive analogue of glucose and studied its uptake in tasks related to vision. The results pointed to the involvement not only of the inferior temporal cortex but also of posterior parietal tissue.

Furthermore, in our laboratory Leslie G. Ungerleider recently found that another anatomical pathway, in addition to the one we now know is devoted to processing the visual characteristics of an object, emerges from the striate cortex (the primary visual station at the back of the brain). Instead of coursing forward into the inferior temporal cortex, this second pathway runs upward through a series of stations to a final station in the posterior parietal cortex. Spatial relations are probably analyzed along this pathway; from its final station processed spatial perceptions presumably activate the subcortical memory system.

The roles of the two memory circuits outlined earlier may differ in spatial learning. Although the hippocampus and the amygdala can substitute for each other in learning to recognize an object, the former structure seems to be particularly important for learning spatial relations. Stimulated by the work of other investigators, whose results had suggested the importance of the hippocampus for spatial learning in rodents, Parkinson explored its role in monkeys.

He trained normal monkeys to perform a test that taxed their memory for the location of objects. In each trial the animals were shown two completely new objects in specific locations on the test tray; next they saw one of the original objects in its original position and an exact duplicate, either where the second object had been or at yet a third position on the tray. The animals were rewarded for choosing the original object in its original position.

After surgery in which their amygdala was removed bilaterally, animals quickly relearned the task and did it accurately. Bilateral removal of the hippocampus, however, left monkeys unable to perform the feat at all. Mary Lou Smith, working with Milner, recently reported a parallel finding in human amnesics: a correlation between the extent of hippocampal damage and the degree of impairment in remembering the locations of objects.

WHERE MEMORY MEETS MEMORY

The amygdala also has its specializations. Many of the amygdala's distinctive contributions to memory were suggested by its remarkable neuroanatomy (see Figure 6.7), which was known long before its role in memory had been established. The amygdala—or, more precisely, the amygdaloid complex, which consists of several nuclei—is a kind of crossroads in the brain. Many investigators, including Blair H. Turner of the Howard University College of Medicine and me, had shown the amygdala has direct and extensive connections with all the sensory systems in the cortex. It also communicates with the thalamus, along a path that is a segment of the memory system. Finally, the same parts of the amygdala on which sensory inputs converge send fibers deeper into the brain to the hypothalamus, which is thought to be the source of emotional responses.

The number and variety of connections between sensory areas and the amygdala led Murray and me to wonder whether it might be responsible for associating memories formed in different senses. Until we turned to that question, we had always investigated learning as it is manifested in recognition, that is, a response to the original visual, tactile or spatial experience. Quite often, however, what awakens a memory is a sensory experience of a different kind. The sound of a familiar voice on the telephone summons a visual memory of the caller's face; the sight of a purple plum brings to mind its taste. Some kind of interchange between the cortical areas where memories in each sense are stored would seem to be necessary for such cross-modal recall. Might it be mediated by the amygdala?

To test the possibility, Murray and I combined visual and tactile versions of the recognition-memory test. We taught monkeys to perform delayed nonmatching-to-sample with objects chosen from a pool of 40, each of them distinctive both visually and tactilely. The animals did the tasks both by sight and in the dark, where they had to rely on their sense of touch to distinguish the sample object

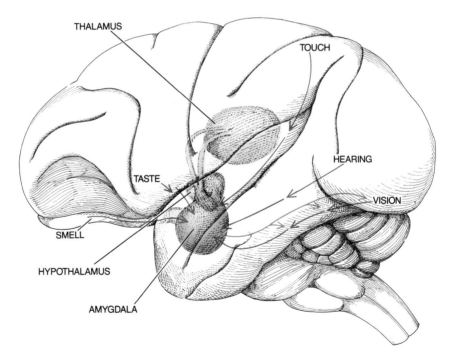

Figure 6.7 MULTIPLE CONNECTIONS of the amygdala underlie the variety of roles it is thought to serve in memory. Fibers reach the amygdala from the final stations of cortical sensory systems (*red arrows*). Sensory impressions thereby activate one circuit of the memory system, which depends on connections (*green*) between the amygdala and the thalamus. Links (*purple*) between the amygdala and the hypothalamus, where emotional responses probably originate, seem to allow an experience to gain emotional associations. Those links may also allow emotions to influence learning, by activating reciprocal connections from the amygdala to sensory paths (*shown in blue, for the visual system only*).

from the new one. Monkeys performed both tasks nearly as well after bilateral removal of the amygdala as they had before the surgery. Their visual and tactile recognition memory had remained largely intact, in keeping with our earlier finding that the hippocampus and the amygdala can substitute for each other in mediating recognition memory.

Now that the monkeys were thoroughly familiar with the visual and tactile qualities of the 40 objects, we changed the nature of the test. In each trial the monkey first examined an object in the dark, by touch, but then confronted the same object and an alternative in the light and had to choose between them by sight alone. To recognize the object it had felt a few seconds earlier, the animal had to associate visual and tactile memories. A control group of animals whose hippocampus had been removed performed the task well, choosing the correct object about 90 percent of the time. Animals lacking their amygdala, on the other hand, did little better than they would have done by chance.

The evidence that the amygdala mediates the association of memories formed through different senses may shed light on an old mystery of neuropsychology. Nearly 50 years ago Heinrich Klüver and P. C. Bucy were struck by the strange behavior of monkeys whose temporal lobes had been removed. The animals often examined an inedible object repeatedly and indiscriminately, by touch, taste and smell, as if they found it perennially unfamiliar. Later the same bizarre effect was shown to follow removal of the amygdala alone. Our result led us to propose that one root of the behavior is the monkeys' inability to link different kinds of memory. Seeing a familiar object, they cannot recall how it smells; after smelling it they still cannot recall its taste.

MIXING MEMORY AND DESIRE

Klüver and Bucy noted another remarkable feature of monkeys lacking temporal lobes, a feature that also was later ascribed to loss of the amygdala. The animals lost their fear of human beings and even their aversion to such normally repugnant sensations as pinching. It was as if a link between familiar stimuli and their emotional associations had been severed. By virtue of its connections with both the sensory areas in the cortex and the triggers of emotional response deep in the brain, the amygdala is

well suited to mediating such a link. The possibility that sensory experiences acquire their emotional weight by way of the amygdala gains support from the observation we made early in the course of our inquiry into memory: monkeys without an amygdala are slow in learning to associate an object with a reward. Such animals have trouble remembering the positive associations of a familiar stimulus.

It is possible that the amygdala not only enables sensory events to develop emotional associations but also enables emotions to shape perception and the storage of memories. How does the brain single out significant stimuli from the welter of impressions supplied by the senses? If emotions can affect sensory processing in the cortex, they might provide the needed filter, tending to limit attention—and hence learning—to stimuli with emotional significance. The amygdala, in its capacity as intermediary between the senses and the emotions, is one structure that could underlie such "selective attention."

Circuitry exists that could give the amygdala this gatekeeping function. Several groups of investigators have established that the sensory systems in the cortex not only send fibers to the amygdala but also receive projections from it—projections that, at least in the visual system, are densest in the highest processing stations. In a collaborative study with Candace B. Pert and others in her laboratory at the National Institute of Mental Health my colleagues and I found a clue to the nature of some of the projections. The amygdala is rich in neurons making opiumlike neurotransmitters known as endogenous opiates, which in other parts of the nervous system are believed to regulate the transmission of nerve signals. We found that the sensory processing pathways in the cortex show a gradient of opiate receptors: the cell-surface molecules to which opiates bind in acting on a neuron. The receptors are most abundant in the final stations, where complete sensory impressions take form.

Together, the evidence suggests the possibility that opiate-containing fibers run from the amygdala to the sensory systems, where they may serve a gatekeeping function by releasing opiates in response to emotional states generated in the hypothalamus. In that way the amygdala may enable the emotions to influence what is perceived and learned. The amygdala's reciprocal effect on the cortex may explain why, in both monkeys and humans, emotionally charged events make a disproportionate impression.

MEMORY AND HABIT

Having mapped two broad circuits, one rooted in the amygdala and the other in the hippocampus, that are responsible for many kinds of cognitive learning—the capacity to recognize a familiar object, recall its unperceived sensory qualities, remember its former location and attach emotional significance to it—we were left with a puzzle. It is embodied in the fact that people suffering from a memory loss so complete that they cannot recognize another person seen just minutes earlier are still capable of learning. Years ago Milner reported that H.M. learned the skill of mirror drawing (drawing while watching one's hand in a mirror). He mastered it at an almost normal rate, even though after he had done so he could not remember ever having performed the feat.

Monkeys whose limbic structures have been destroyed can also learn. Such animals are helpless when it comes to the delayed nonmatching-to-sample test, in which they must recognize an object seen just once. Yet in our laboratory Barbara L. Malamut has found that if a long series of different object pairs, each containing one baited object, is shown to the same monkeys just once a day, with time they learn to choose the object carrying the reward. What is more, they gain facility at about the same rate as normal monkeys. To a human observer the second task seems, if anything, harder than the first one. How can one reconcile these seemingly contradictory results?

Like many other investigators of memory mechanisms, I have argued for the existence of a second system of learning, one that is independent of the limbic circuits. It is a system for which the critical element is stimulus-response repetition—exactly what is missing in delayed nonmatching-to-sample. In keeping with the evidence from human amnesics, Herbert L. Petri and I have proposed that the second system yields a different kind of learning from the memories stored by way of the limbic circuits.

We call this kind of learning "habit." It is noncognitive: it is founded not on knowledge or even on memories (in the sense of independent mental entities) but on automatic connections between a stimulus and a response. In the object-discrimination test the monkey confronts the same pair of stimuli day after day; eventually it develops a habit of picking the object whose selection is always reinforced with a reward. The nonmatching-to-sample task, on the other hand, cannot be satisfied by habit formation. The stimulus to be remembered is shown only once, and the monkey must then respond not to the same stimulus—the one that first carried the reward—but to a new one. It must know, in a cognitive sense, which of the objects is the original one in order to avoid it.

Habits, as we define them, are reminiscent of the automatic stimulus-response bonds that behaviorist psychologists long ago argued are the basis of all learning. The behaviorist point of view excludes such terms as "mind," "knowledge" and even "memory," in its usual sense. It stands in opposition to cognitive psychology, which relies on those very concepts to account for much of behavior. The possibility that learning is built on two quite different systems, one of them a source of noncognitive habits and the other the basis of cognitive memory, offers a way to reconcile the behaviorist and cognitivist schools. If neural mechanisms for both kinds of learning do exist, behavior could be a blend of automatic responses to stimuli and actions guided by knowledge and expectation.

A likely neural substrate for habit formation is the striatum, a complex of structures in the forebrain (see Figure 6.8). The striatum receives projections from many areas of the cortex, including the sensory systems, and sends fibers to the parts of the brain that control movement. Hence it is neuroanatomically suited to providing the relatively direct links between stimulus and action that are implicit in the notion of habit. Indeed, other workers have found that damage to the striatum impairs the ability of monkeys to form habits of the kind that are tested in the object-discrimination task.

Paul D. MacLean of the National Institute of Mental Health has pointed out that the striatum is an evolutionarily ancient part of the brain, older by far than the cortex and the limbic system. One would expect habit formation to be mediated by primitive structures: even simple animals can learn automatic responses to stimuli. Developmentally, habit seems to be primitive as well. Bachevalier has recently found that infant monkeys do about as well as adults on our test of habit formation, and yet they do poorly on the memory test. By adult standards they are amnesic. We are now looking into the possibility that the neural substrate of habit is fully developed in infant monkeys, whereas the memory system is slow to mature. The same devel-

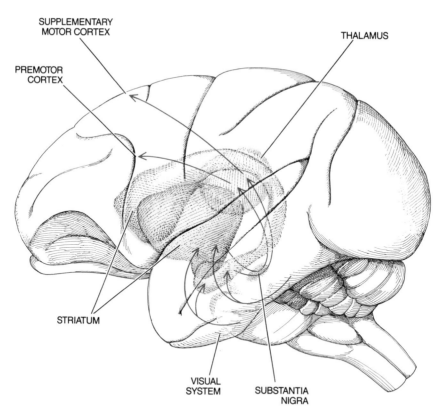

SUPPLEMENTARY
MOTOR CORTEX

PREMOTOR
CORTEX

THALAMUS

STRIATUM

VISUAL
SYSTEM

SUBSTANTIA
NIGRA

Figure 6.8 HABIT FORMATION, or the development of automatic connections between a stimulus and a response, may depend on the striatum. It receives extensive connections from sensory systems in the cortex (here typified by one branch of the visual system) and in turn sends fibers to cerebral structures that communicate with the premotor cortex and the supplementary motor cortex. The neuroanatomy thus provides a relatively direct path through which a stimulus registered in a sensory area could lead to a motor response. Indeed, damage to the striatum or to connections between the cortex and the striatum has been found to hamper monkeys' performance on a visual test measuring habit formation.

opmental difference, if it is present in human beings, could explain why few people remember their infancy.

As for how memory and habit interact in the mature brain, we are only starting to formulate our questions. It seems likely that most kinds of learning draw on both systems, but it is easy to see that cognitive memory and noncognitive habit would often conflict. How does the brain adjudicate between habit formation and cognitive learning? Do elements of the memory system communicate with the striatum and thereby influence habit formation? In surveying the cerebral territory of memory and habit we have only mapped a landscape for future exploration.

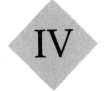

OF SYMMETRY, IMAGINING AND DREAMING

. . .

Specializations of the Human Brain

Certain higher faculties, such as language, depend on specialized regions in the human brain. On a larger scale the two cerebral hemispheres are specialized for different kinds of mental activity.

• • •

Norman Geschwind
September, 1979

The nervous systems of all animals have a number of basic functions in common, most notably the control of movement and the analysis of sensation. What distinguishes the human brain is the variety of more specialized activities it is capable of learning. The preeminent example is language: no one is born knowing a language, but virtually everyone learns to speak and to understand the spoken word, and people of all cultures can be taught to write and to read. Music is also universal in man: people with no formal training are able to recognize and to reproduce dozens of melodies. Similarly, almost everyone can draw simple figures, and the ability to make accurate renderings is not rare.

At least some of these higher functions of the human brain are governed by dedicated networks of neurons. It has been known for more than 100 years, for example, that at least two delimited regions of the cerebral cortex are essential to linguistic competence; they seem to be organized explicitly for the processing of verbal information. Certain structures on the inner surface of the underside of the temporal lobe, including the hippocampus, are apparently necessary for the long-term retention of memories. In some cases the functional specializa-

tion of a neural system seems to be quite narrowly defined: hence one area on both sides of the human cerebral cortex is concerned primarily with the recognition of faces. It is likely that other mental activities are also associated with particular neural networks. Musical and artistic abilities, for example, appear to depend on specialized systems in the brain, although the circuitry has not yet been worked out.

Another distinctive characteristic of the human brain is the allocation of functions to the two cerebral hemispheres. That the human brain is not fully symmetrical in its functioning could be guessed from at least one observation of daily experience: most of the human population favors the right hand, which is controlled by the left side of the brain. Linguistic abilities also reside mainly on the left side. For these reasons the left cerebral hemisphere was once said to be the dominant one and the right side of the brain was thought to be subservient. In recent years this concept has been revised as it has become apparent that each hemisphere has its own specialized talents. Those for which the right cortex is dominant include some features of aptitudes for music and for the recognition of complex visual patterns. The right hemisphere is also the more important one for the expression and recognition of emotion. In the past few years these functional asymmetries have been matched with anatomical ones, and a start has been made on exploring their prevalence in species other than man.

In man as in other mammalian species large areas of the cerebral cortex are given over to comparatively elementary sensory and motor functions. An arch that extends roughly from ear to ear across the roof of the brain is the primary motor cortex, which exercises voluntary control over the muscles. Parallel to this arch and just behind it is the primary somatic sensory area, where signals are received from the skin, the bones, the joints and the muscles. Almost every region of the body is represented by a corresponding region in both the primary motor cortex and the somatic sensory cortex. At the back of the brain, and particularly on the inner surface of the occipital lobes, is the primary visual cortex. The primary auditory areas are in the temporal lobes; olfaction is focused in a region on the underside of the frontal lobes.

The primary motor and sensory areas are specialized in the sense that each one is dedicated to a specified function, but the functions themselves are of general utility, and the areas are called on in a great variety of activities (see Figure 7.1). Moreover, homologous areas are found in all species that have a well-developed cerebral cortex. My main concern in this article is with certain regions of the cortex that govern a narrower range of behavior. Some of

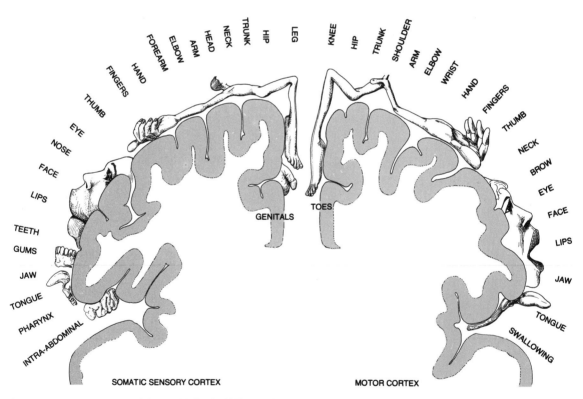

Figure 7.1 SOMATIC SENSORY AND MOTOR REGIONS of the cerebral cortex are specialized in the sense that every site in these regions can be associated with some part of the body. In other words, most of the body can be mapped onto the cortex, yielding two distorted homunculi. The distortions come about because the area of the cortex dedicated to a part of the body is proportional not to that part's actual size but to the precision with which it must be controlled. In man the motor and somatic sensory regions given over to the face and to the hands are greatly exaggerated. Only half of each cortical region is shown: the left somatic sensory area (which receives sensations primarily from the right side of the body) and the right motor cortex (which exercises control over movement in the left half of the body).

these highly specialized areas may be common to many species but others may be uniquely human.

A series of experiments dealing with learning in monkeys illustrates how fine the functional distinction can be between two networks of neurons. A monkey can be taught to choose consistently one object or pattern from a pair. The task is made somewhat more difficult if the objects are presented and then withdrawn and the monkey is allowed to indicate its choice only after a delay during which the objects are hidden behind a screen. It has been found that performance on this test is impaired markedly if a small region of the frontal lobes is destroyed on both sides of the brain. Difficulty can also be introduced into the experiment by making the patterns complex but allowing a choice to be made while the patterns are still in sight. Damage to a quite different area of the cortex reduces ability to carry out this task, but it has no effect on the delay test.

These experiments also illustrate one of the principal means for acquiring information about the functions of the brain. When a particular site is damaged by disease or injury, a well-defined deficiency in behavior sometimes ensues. In many cases one may conclude that some aspects of the behavior affected are normally dependent on the part of the brain that has been destroyed. In man the commonest cause of brain damage is cerebral thrombosis, or stroke: the occlusion of arteries in the brain, which results in the death of the tissues the blocked arteries supply. By 1920 the study of patients who had sustained such damage had led to the identification of several functional regions of the brain, including the language areas.

The study of the effects of damage to the brain is still an important method of investigating brain function, but other techniques have since been developed. One of the most important was brought to a high level of development by the German neurosurgeon Otfrid Foerster and by Wilder Penfield of the Montreal Neurological Institute. They studied the responses in the conscious patient undergoing brain surgery that follow electrical stimulation of various sites in the brain. In this way they were able to map the regions responsible for a number of functions. Apart from the importance of this technique for the study of the brain, it is of clinical benefit since it enables the surgeon to avoid areas where damage might be crippling.

Surgical procedures developed for the control of severe epilepsy have also contributed much information. One method of treating persistent epileptic seizures (adopted only when other therapies have failed) is to remove the region of the cortex from which the seizures arise. The functional deficits that sometimes result from this procedure have been studied in detail by Brenda Milner of the Montreal Neurological Institute.

The specializations of the hemispheres can be studied in people who have sustained damage to the commissures that connect the two sides of the brain, the most important of these being the corpus callosum. In the first such cases, studied at the end of the 19th century by Jules Déjerine in France and by Hugo Liepmann in Germany, the damage had been caused by strokes. More recently isolation of the hemispheres by surgical sectioning of the commissures has been employed for the relief of epilepsy. Studies of such "split brain" patients (see Figure 7.2) by Roger W. Sperry of the California Institute of Technology and by Michael S. Gazzaniga of the Cornell University Medical College have provided increasingly detailed knowledge of the functions of the separated hemispheres. Doreen Kimura, who is now at the University of Western Ontario, pioneered in the development of a technique, called dichotic listening, that provides information about hemispheric specialization in the intact human brain.

The specialized regions of the brain that have been investigated in the greatest detail are those involved in language. In the 1860's the French investigator Paul Broca pointed out that damage to a particular region of the cortex consistently gives rise to an aphasia, or speech disorder. The region is on the side of the frontal lobes, and it is now called the anterior language area, or simply Broca's area. Broca went on to make a second major discovery. He showed that whereas damage to this area on the left side of the brain leads to aphasia, similar damage to the corresponding area on the right side leaves the faculty of speech intact. This finding has since been amply confirmed: well over 95 percent of the aphasias caused by brain damage result from damage to the left hemisphere.

Broca's area is adjacent to the face area of the motor cortex, which controls the muscles of the face, the tongue, the jaw and the throat (see Figure 7.3). When Broca's area is destroyed by a stroke, there is almost always severe damage to the face area in the left hemisphere as well, and so it might be thought that the disruption of speech is caused

REPRODUCED BY LEFT HAND
(RIGHT HEMISPHERE)

MODEL PATTERN

REPRODUCED BY RIGHT HAND
(LEFT HEMISPHERE)

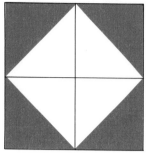
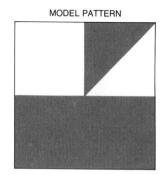
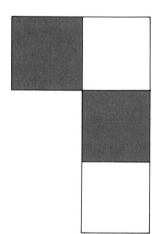

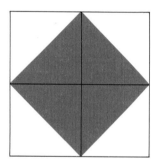

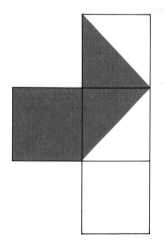

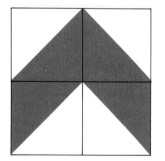

Figure 7.2 TWO HEMISPHERES of the human cerebral cortex were tested in a subject whose hemispheres had been surgically isolated from each other. Each of the patterns in the middle column was presented to the subject, who was asked to reproduce it by assembling colored blocks, either with the right hand alone (which communicates mainly with the left hemisphere) or with the left hand alone (controlled primarily by the right hemisphere). Errors were equally frequent with either hand, but the kinds of error typical of each hand were quite different. The results suggest that each side of the brain may bring a separate set of skills to bear on such a task. (Test was conducted by Edith Kaplan at the Boston Veterans Administration Hospital).

by partial paralysis of the muscles required for articulation. That some other explanation is required is easily demonstrated. First, damage to the corresponding area on the right side of the brain does not cause aphasia, although a similar weakness of the facial muscles results. Furthermore, in Broca's aphasia it is known that the muscles that function poorly in speech operate normally in other tasks. The evidence is quite simple: the patient with Broca's aphasia can speak only with great difficulty, but he can sing with ease and often with elegance. The speech of a patient with Broca's aphasia also has features, such as faulty grammar, that cannot be explained by a muscular failure.

Another kind of aphasia was identified in 1874 by the German investigator Carl Wernicke. It is associated with damage to another site in the cortex, also in the left hemisphere, but in the temporal lobe rather than the frontal lobe. This region, which is now called Wernicke's area, lies between the primary auditory cortex and a structure called the angular gyrus (see Figure 7.3), which probably mediates between visual and auditory centers of the brain. It has since been learned that Wernicke's area and Broca's area are connected by a bundle of nerve fibers, the arcuate fasciculus.

A lesion in either Broca's area or Wernicke's area leads to a disruption of speech, but the nature of the two disorders is quite different. In Broca's aphasia speech is labored and slow and articulation is impaired. The response to a question will often make sense, but it generally cannot be expressed as a fully formed or grammatical sentence. There is particular difficulty with the inflection of verbs, with pronouns and connective words and with complex grammatical constructions. As a result the speech has a telegraphic style. For example, a pa-

tient asked about a dental appointment said, hesitantly and indistinctly: "Yes . . . Monday . . . Dad and Dick . . . Wednesday nine o'clock . . . 10 o'clock . . . doctors . . . and . . . teeth." The same kinds of errors are made in writing.

In Wernicke's aphasia speech is phonetically and even grammatically normal, but it is semantically deviant. Words are often strung together with considerable facility and with the proper inflections, so that the utterance has the recognizable structure of a sentence. The words chosen, however, are often inappropriate, and they sometimes include nonsensical syllables or words. Even when the individual words are correct, the utterance as a whole may express its meaning in a remarkably roundabout way. A patient who was asked to describe a picture that showed two boys stealing cookies behind a woman's back reported: "Mother is away here working her work to get her better, but when she's looking the two boys looking in the other part. She's working another time."

From an analysis of these defects Wernicke formulated a model of language production in the brain. Much new information has been added in the past 100 years, but the general principles Wernicke elaborated still seem valid. In this model the underlying structure of an utterance arises in Wernicke's area. It is then transferred through the arcuate fasciculus to Broca's area, where it evokes a detailed and coordinated program for vocalization. The program is passed on to the adjacent face area of the motor cortex, which activates the appropriate muscles of the mouth, the lips, the tongue, the larynx and so on.

Wernicke's area not only has a part in speaking but also has a major role in the comprehension of the spoken word and in reading and writing (see Figure 7.4). When a word is heard, the sound is initially received in the primary auditory cortex, but the signal must pass through the adjacent Wernicke's area if it is to be understood as a verbal message. When a word is read, the visual pattern (from the primary visual cortex) is transmitted to the angular gyrus, which applies a transformation that elicits the auditory form of the word in Wernicke's area. Writing a word in response to an oral instruction requires information to be passed along the same pathways in the opposite direction: from the auditory cortex to Wernicke's area to the angular gyrus.

This model explains many of the symptoms that

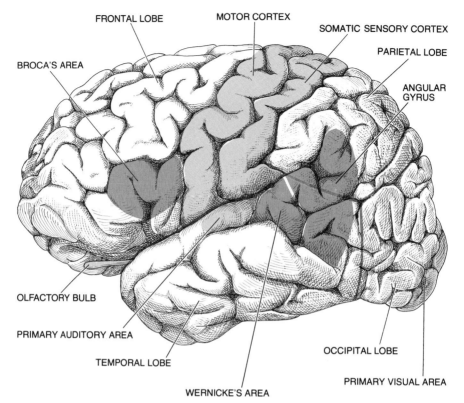

FRONTAL LOBE

MOTOR CORTEX

SOMATIC SENSORY CORTEX

PARIETAL LOBE

BROCA'S AREA

ANGULAR GYRUS

OLFACTORY BULB

PRIMARY AUDITORY AREA

TEMPORAL LOBE

OCCIPITAL LOBE

PRIMARY VISUAL AREA

WERNICKE'S AREA

Figure 7.3 MAP OF THE HUMAN CORTEX shows regions whose functional specializations have been identified. These areas, which include the motor and somatic sensory regions and the primary visual, auditory and olfactory areas, are present in all species that have a well-developed cortex. Several other regions (*dark color*) are more narrowly specialized. These functional specializations have been detected only on the left side of the brain. The right hemisphere (not shown) has its own specialized abilities. The assignment of functions to sites in the left hemisphere is only approximate; some areas may have functions in addition to those indicated, and some functions may be carried out in more than one place.

characterize the aphasias. A lesion in Broca's area disturbs the production of speech but has a much smaller effect on comprehension. Damage to Wernicke's area, on the other hand, disrupts all aspects of the use of language. The effects of certain rarer lesions are also in accord with the model. For example, destruction of the arcuate fasciculus, disconnecting Wernicke's area from Broca's area, leaves speech fluent and well articulated but semantically aberrant; Broca's area is operating but it is not receiving information from Wernicke's area. Because the latter center is also functional, however, comprehension of spoken and written words is almost normal. Writing is disrupted in all aphasias where speech is abnormal, but the neural circuits employed in writing are not known in detail.

Lesions in the angular gyrus have the effect of disconnecting the systems involved in auditory language and written language. Patients with injuries in certain areas of the angular gyrus may speak and understand speech normally, but they have difficulty with written language. The comprehension of a written word seems to require that the auditory form of the word be evoked in Wernicke's area. Damage to the angular gyrus seems to interrupt communication between the visual cortex and Wernicke's area, so that comprehension of written language is impaired.

Although the partitioning of linguistic functions among several sites in the cortex is now supported by much evidence, the rigidity of these assignments should not be overemphasized. The pessimistic

SPEAKING A HEARD WORD

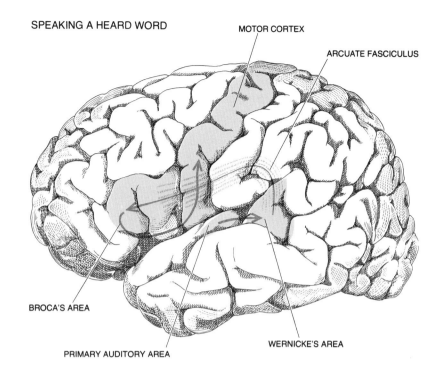

Figure 7.4 LINGUISTIC COMPE-TENCE. When a word is heard (*top*) the sensation from the ears is received by the primary auditory cortex, but the word cannot be understood until the signal is processed in Wernicke's area. If the word is to be spoken, some representation of it is thought to be transmitted to Broca's area, where the word evokes a detailed program for articulation, which is supplied to the motor cortex, which drives the muscles of the lips, tongue, larynx and so on. When a written word is read (*bottom*) the sensation is registered by the primary visual cortex. It is then thought to be relayed to the angular gyrus, which associates the visual form of the word with the corresponding auditory pattern in Wernicke's area.

view that damage to tissue in these areas inevitably leads to a permanent linguistic impairment is unwarranted (see Figure 7.5). Actually a considerable degree of recovery is often observed. The neural tissue destroyed by an arterial thrombosis cannot be regenerated, but it seems the functions of the damaged areas can often be assumed, at least in part, by other regions. In some cases the recovery probably reflects the existence of an alternative store of learning on the opposite side of the brain, which remains dormant until the dominant side is injured. In other cases the function is taken over by neurons in areas adjacent to or surrounding the damaged site. Patrick D. Wall of University College London has shown that there is a fringe of such dormant but potentially active cells adjacent to the somatic sensory cortex, and it seems likely that similar fringe regions exist throughout the brain. Jay P. Mohr and his co-workers have shown that the prospects for recovery from Broca's aphasia are quite good provided the region destroyed is not too large. One interpretation

of these findings suggests that regions bordering on Broca's area share its specialization in latent form.

Although the detailed mechanism of recovery is not known, it has been established that some groups of patients are more likely than others to regain their linguistic competence. Children, particularly children younger than eight, often make an excellent recovery. Left-handed people also make better progress than right-handers. Even among right-handers those who have left-handed parents, siblings or children are more likely to recover than those with no family history of left-handedness. The relation between handedness and recovery from damage to the language areas suggests that cerebral dominance for handedness and dominance for language are not totally independent.

A disorder of the brain that is startling because its effects are so narrowly circumscribed is prosopagnosia; it is a failure to recognize faces. In the normal individual the ability to identify people from

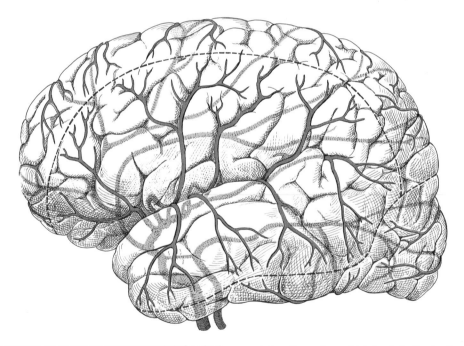

Figure 7.5 VASCULAR SYSTEM OF THE BRAIN has had an important part in the mapping of functional regions in the cerebral cortex. The normal functions of an area can often be inferred from the disturbance or impairment of behavior that results when the area is damaged. The commonest cause of such damage is the occlusion of an artery supplying the cortex, which leads to the death of the tissue nourished by that artery. Broca's area and Wernicke's area were identified in this way about 100 years ago, when patients with distinctive aphasias, or speech defects, were found by postmortem examination to have damage in those areas of the left hemisphere.

their faces is itself quite remarkable. At a glance one can name a person from facial features alone, even though the features may change substantially over the years or may be presented in a highly distorted form, as in a caricature. In a patient with prosopagnosia this talent for association is abolished (see Figure 7.6).

What is most remarkable about the disorder is its specificity. In general it is accompanied by few other neurological symptoms except for the loss of some part of the visual field, sometimes on both sides and sometimes only in the left half of space. Most mental tasks, including those that require the processing of visual information, are done without particular difficulty; for example, the patient can usually read and correctly name seen objects. What he cannot do is look at a person or at a photograph of a face and name the person. He may even fail to recognize his wife or his children. It is not the iden-

tity of familiar people that has been lost to him, however, but only the connection between the face and the identity. When a familiar person speaks, the patient knows the voice and can say the name immediately. The perception of facial features is also unimpaired, since the patient can often describe a face in detail and can usually match a photograph made from the front with a profile of the same person. The deficiency seems to be confined to forming associations between faces and identities.

The lesions that cause prosopagnosia are as stereotyped as the disorder itself. Damage is found on the underside of both occipital lobes, extending forward to the inner surface of the temporal lobes. The implication is that some neural network within this region is specialized for the rapid and reliable recognition of human faces. It may seem that a disproportionate share of the brain's resources is being devoted to a rather limited task. It should be kept in

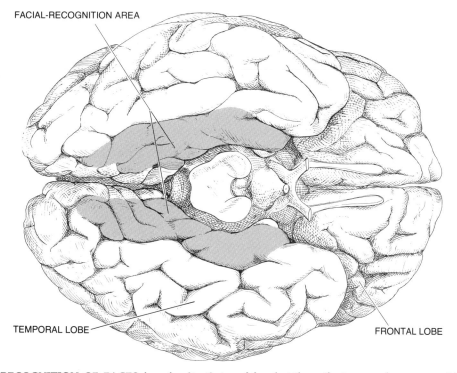

FACIAL-RECOGNITION AREA

TEMPORAL LOBE

FRONTAL LOBE

Figure 7.6 RECOGNITION OF FACES is a faculty that seems to be governed by regions on the underside of the temporal and occipital lobes on both sides of the cortex, seen here from below. A lesion that destroys this area impairs the ability to identify a person by facial features but has almost no other effects. There is often some loss of vision, but the patient can read, can name objects on sight and can even match a full-face portrait with a profile of the same person. People can also be recognized by their voices. The only ability that is lost is the ability to recognize people by their faces, and that loss can be so severe that close relatives are not recognized.

mind, however, that the recognition of people as individuals is a valuable talent in a highly social animal, and there has probably been strong selectional pressure to improve its efficiency.

Similar capacities probably exist in other social species. Gary W. Van Hoesen, formerly in my department at the Harvard Medical School and now at the University of Iowa College of Medicine, has begun to investigate the neurological basis of face recognition in the rhesus monkey. So far he has demonstrated that the monkeys can readily discriminate between other monkeys on the basis of facial photographs. The neural structures called into play by this task have not, however, been identified.

Until recently little was known about the physiological basis of memory, one of the most important functions of the human brain. Through the study of some highly specific disorders, however, it has been possible to identify areas or structures in the brain that are involved in certain memory processes. For example, the examination of different forms of anterograde amnesia—an inability to learn new information—has revealed the role of the temporal lobes in memory. In particular, the striking disability of a patient whom Milner has studied for more than 25 years demonstrates the importance in memory of structures on the inner surface of the temporal lobes, such as the hippocampus (see Figure 7.7).

In 1953 the patient had submitted to a radical surgical procedure in which much of the hippocampus and several associated structures in both temporal lobes were destroyed. After the operation the skills and knowledge the patient had acquired up to that time remained largely intact, and he was and still is able to attend normally to ongoing events. In fact, he seems to be able to register limited amounts of new information in the usual manner. Within a short time, however, most of the newly learned information ceases to be available to him.

Milner has interviewed and tested the patient at intervals since the operation, and she has found that his severe anterograde amnesia has changed very little during that time. She has also exhibited an extensive although patchy retrograde amnesia (about the years before the operation), but that has improved appreciably. In the absence of distraction he can retain, say, a three-digit number for many minutes by means of verbal rehearsal or with the aid of an elaborate mnemonic device. Once his attention has been momentarily diverted, however, he cannot remember the number or the mnemonic device to which he devoted so much effort. He cannot even remember the task itself. Living from moment to moment, he has not been able to learn his address or to remember where the objects he uses every day are kept in his home. He fails to recognize people who have visited him regularly for many years.

The bilateral surgery that resulted in this memory impairment is, for obvious reasons, no longer done, but similar lesions on the inner surface of the temporal lobes have occasionally resulted from operations on one side of the brain in a patient with unsuspected damage to the opposite lobe. Comparable memory deficits result, and so the role of the inner surface of the temporal lobes in memory function is now widely accepted. Moreover, the fact that these patients generally retain their faculties of perception supports the distinction made by many workers between a short-term memory process and a long-term process by which more stable storage of information is achieved. It is clearly the second process that is impaired in the patients described above, but the nature of the impairment is a matter of controversy. Some think the problem is a failure of consolidation, that is, transferring information from short-term to long-term storage. Others hold that the information is transferred and stored but cannot be retrieved. The ultimate resolution of these conflicting theories will require a clearer specification of the neural circuitry of memory.

At a glance the brain appears to have perfect bilateral symmetry, like most other organs of the body. It might therefore be expected that the two halves of the brain would also be functionally equivalent, just as the two kidneys or the two lungs are. Actually many of the more specialized functions are found in only one hemisphere or the other. Even the apparent anatomical symmetry turns out to be illusory.

In the primary motor and sensory areas of the cortex the assignment of duties to the two hemispheres follows a simple pattern: each side of the brain is concerned mainly with the opposite side of the body. Most of the nerve fibers in the pathways that radiate from the motor and somatic sensory areas cross to the opposite side of the nervous system at some point in their course. Hence the muscles of the right hand and foot are controlled primarily by the left motor cortex, and sensory

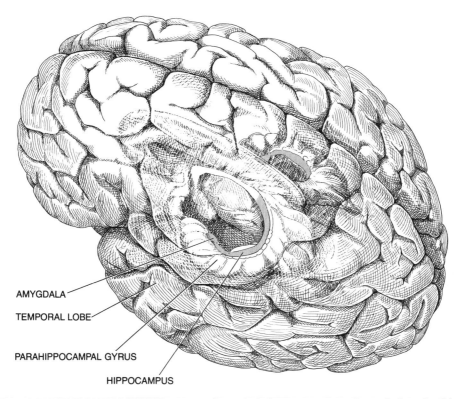

AMYGDALA

TEMPORAL LOBE

PARAHIPPOCAMPAL GYRUS

HIPPOCAMPUS

Figure 7.7 CERTAIN MEMORY PROCESSES appear to be associated with structures on the inner surface of the temporal lobes, such as the hippocampus (*color*). Bilateral lesions of these areas have been shown to cause a severe and lasting memory disorder. Patients with lesions of this type appear to have undiminished powers of perception but are largely incapable of incorporating new information into their long-term store. Acute lesions in this region of a single temporal lobe sometimes result in similar but less persistent memory disorders that reflect the contrasting specializations of the hemispheres: the type of information that cannot be learned varies according to the side the lesion is on.

impulses from the right side go mainly to the left somatic sensory cortex. Each ear has connections to the auditory cortex on both sides of the brain, but the connections to the contralateral side are stronger. The distribution of signals from the eyes is somewhat more complicated. The optic nerves are arranged so that images from the right half of space in both eyes are projected onto the left visual cortex; the left visual field from both eyes goes to the right hemisphere. As a result of this pattern of contralateral connections the sensory and motor functions of the two hemispheres are kept separate, but the are largely symmetrical. Each half of the brain is concerned with half of the body and half of the visual field.

The distribution of the more specialized functions is quite different, and it is profoundly asymmetrical.

I have indicated above that linguistic ability is dependent primarily on the left hemisphere. There is reason to believe the right side of the brain is more important for the perception of melodies, one item of evidence being the ease with which aphasic patients with left-hemisphere damage can sing. The perception and analysis of nonverbal visual patterns, such as perspective drawings, is largely a function of the right hemisphere, although the left hemisphere also makes a distinctive contribution to such tasks. These asymmetries are also reflected in partial memory defects that can result from lesions in a single temporal lobe. A left temporal lobectomy can impair the ability to retain verbal material but can leave intact the ability to remember spatial locations, faces, melodies and abstract visual patterns.

In everyday life this lateralization of function can

seldom be detected because information is readily passed between the hemispheres through several commissures, including the corpus callosum. Even when the interconnections are severed, the full effects of cerebral dominance can be observed only in laboratory situations, where it is possible to ensure that sensory information reaches only one hemisphere at a time and that a motor response comes from only one hemisphere. Under these conditions a remarkable pattern of behavior is observed. If an object is placed in a patient's left hand or if it is presented only to his left visual field, he cannot say its name. The failure is not one of recognition, since the patient is able to match related objects, but the perception received only in the right hemisphere cannot be associated with a name that is known only to the left hemisphere.

The specialization of the isolated hemispheres should not be overstated, however. The right half of the brain does have some rudimentary linguistic ability. Moreover, there are doubtless many tasks where the two hemispheres ordinarily act in concert. In one test administered after surgical isolation of the hemispheres the patient is asked to reproduce a simple pattern by assembling colored blocks. In some cases errors are frequent whether the task is completed with the left hand or the right, but they are characteristically different kinds of errors. It appears that neither hemisphere alone is competent in this task and that the two must cooperate.

One of the most surprising recent findings is that different emotional reactions follow damage to the right and left sides of the brain. Lesions in most areas on the left side are accompanied by the feelings of loss that might be expected as a result of any serious injury. The patient is disturbed by his disability and often is depressed. Damage in much of the right hemisphere sometimes leaves the patient unconcerned with his condition. Guido Gainotti in Rome has made a detailed compilation of these differences in emotional response.

Emotion and "state of mind" are often associated with the structures of the limbic system, at the core of the brain, but in recent years it has been recognized that the cerebral cortex, particularly the right hemisphere of the cortex, also makes an important contribution. Lesions in the right hemisphere not only give rise to inappropriate emotional responses to the patient's own condition but also impair his recognition of emotion in others. A patient with damage on the left side may not be able to comprehend a statement, but in many cases he can still recognize the emotional tone with which it is spoken. A patient with a disorder of the right hemisphere usually understands the meaning of what is said, but he often fails to recognize that it is spoken in an angry or a humorous way.

Although cerebral dominance has been known in the human brain for more than a century, comparable asymmetries in other species have been recognized only in the past few years. A pioneer in this endeavor is Fernando Nottebohm of Rockefeller University, who has studied the neural basis of singing in songbirds. In most of the species he has studied so far, but not in all of them, the left side of the brain is more important for singing. Examples of dominance in mammals other than man have also been described, although in much less detail. Under certain conditions damage to the right side of the brain in rats alters emotional behavior, as Victor H. Denenberg of the University of Connecticut has shown. Dominance of the left cerebral cortex for some auditory tasks has been discovered in one species of monkey by James H. Dewson III. Michael Petersen and other investigators at the University of Michigan and at Rockefeller University have shown that the left hemisphere is dominant in the recognition of species-specific cries in Japanese macaques, which employ an unusual variety of such signals. So far, however, no definitive example of functional asymmetry has been described in the brains of the great apes, the closest relations of man.

For many years it was the prevailing view of neurologists that the functional asymmetries of the brain could not be correlated with anatomical asymmetries. If there were any significant differences between the hemispheres, it was assumed, they would have been noted long ago by surgeons or pathologists. About 10 years ago my colleague Walter Levitsky and I decided to look into this matter again, following some earlier observations by the German neurologist Richard Arwed Pfeifer. We examined 100 human brains, paying particular attention to a region called the planum temporale, which lies on the upper surface of the temporal lobe and is hidden within the sylvian fissure that runs along each side of the brain (see Figure 7.8). Our study was concerned only with gross anatomy, and we employed no instruments more elaborate than a camera and a ruler; nevertheless, we found unequivocal evidence of asymmetry. In general the

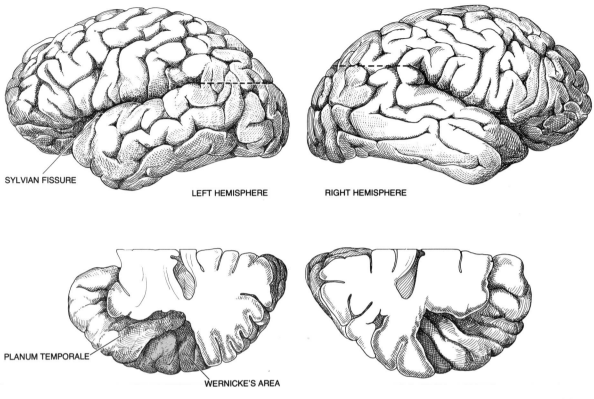

SYLVIAN FISSURE

LEFT HEMISPHERE   RIGHT HEMISPHERE

PLANUM TEMPORALE

WERNICKE'S AREA

Figure 7.8 ANATOMICAL ASYMMETRY of the cortex has been detected in the human brain and may be related to the distinctive functional specializations of the two hemispheres. One asymmetry is observed in the sylvian fissure, which defines the upper margin of the temporal lobe and rises more steeply on the right side of the brain. A more striking asymmetry is found on the planum tempor-ale, which forms the upper surface of the temporal lobe, and which can be seen only when the sylvian fissure is opened. The posterior part of the planum temporale is usually much larger on the left side. The enlarged region is part of Wernicke's area, suggesting that the asymmetry may be related to the linguistic dominance of the left hemisphere.

length and orientation of the sylvian fissures is different on opposite sides of the head. What is more significant, the posterior area of the planum temporale, which forms part of Wernicke's area, is generally larger on the left side. The differences are not subtle and can easily be seen with the unaided eye.

Juhn A. Wada of the University of British Columbia subsequently showed that the asymmetry of the planum temporale can be detected in the human fetus. It therefore appears that the enlargement of the left planum cannot be a response to the development of linguistic competence in childhood. On the contrary, the superior linguistic talent of the left hemisphere may result from the anatomical bias.

More recently my colleague Albert M. Galaburda has discovered that the enlargement of the left planum can be explained in terms of the cellular organization of the tissue. On the planum is a region with a distinctive cellular architecture, designated *Tpt*. Galaburda found that the extent of the *Tpt* region is considerably greater in the left hemisphere; in the first brain he examined it was more than seven times as large on the left side as it was on the right.

Galaburda and Thomas Kemper, working at the Boston University School of Medicine, also examined the brain of an accident victim who had suffered from persistent dyslexia (see Figure 7.9). He

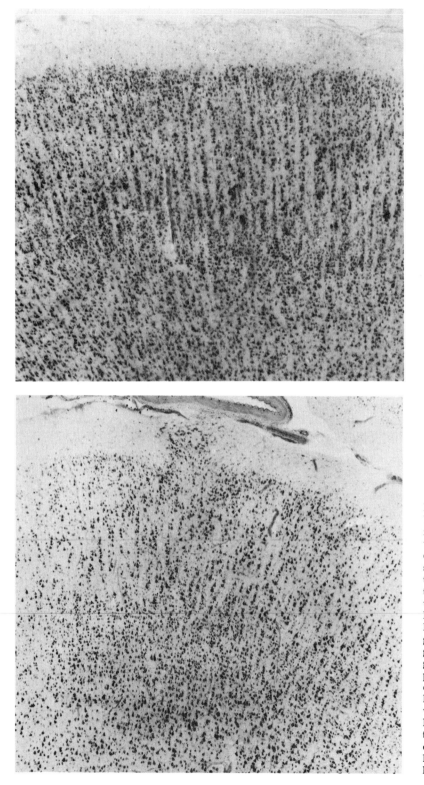

Figure 7.9 ABNORMAL CELLU-LAR ARCHITECTURE has been found in a language area of a patient with a developmental reading dis-order. The top photomicrograph is a section of the normal cortex from the posterior portion of the planum temporale, the region that makes up part of Wernicke's area. Several layers can be perceived and the cells have a characteristic columnar or-ganization. The bottom micro-graph is a section from the same re-gion in a patient with dyslexia. One peculiarity is the presence of nerve-cell bodies in the most superficial layer (*near top of micrograph*), where they are normally absent. Moreover, throughout the tissue the arrangement of cells is disrupted. (Micrographs by Albert M. Galaburda and Thomas Kemper.)

found that the *Tpt* areas in the two hemispheres were of approximately equal size. Furthermore, the cellular structure of the *Tpt* area on the left side was abnormal. The neurons in the normal cortex are arranged in a sequence of layers, each of which has a distinctive population of cells. In the brain of the dyslexic the strata were disrupted, one conspicuous anomaly being the presence of cell bodies of neurons in the most superficial layer of the cortex, where they are normally absent. Islands of cortical tissue were also found in the white matter of the brain, where they do not belong. Although no firm conclusion can be drawn from a single case, it does seem striking that a structural abnormality would be found in the language area of a patient who was known to have a linguistic disability.

A new line of research on brain asymmetry has lately been opened by my colleague Marjorie J. LeMay. She has devised several methods for detecting anatomical asymmetry in the living person. One of these methods is cerebral arteriography, in which a substance opaque to X rays is injected into the bloodstream and the distribution of the substance is monitored as it flows through the cranial arteries. Arteriography is often employed in the diagnosis of brain tumors and other brain diseases, and the arteriograms LeMay examined had been made for diagnostic purposes. One of the cranial arteries (the middle cerebral artery) follows the groove of the sylvian fissure, and LeMay showed that the position of the artery in the arteriogram reveals the length and orientation of the fissure. She found that in most people the middle cerebral artery on the right side of the head is inclined more steeply and ultimately ascends higher than the corresponding artery on the left side.

LeMay has also detected brain asymmetries by computed axial tomography, the process whereby an image of the skull in cross section is reconstructed from a set of X-ray projections. In these images a peculiar, skewed departure from bilateral symmetry is observed. In right-handed people the right frontal lobe is usually wider than the left, but the left parietal and occipital lobes are wider than the right. The inner surface of the skull itself bulges at the right front and the left rear to accommodate the protuberances.

LeMay has even reported finding asymmetries in cranial endocasts made from the fossil skulls of Neanderthal man and other hominids. A ridge on the inner surface of the skull corresponds to the sylvian fissure; where the ridge is preserved well enough to make an impression in an endocast LeMay finds the same pattern of asymmetry that is observed in modern man, suggesting that hemispheric dominance had already emerged at least 30,000 years ago. LeMay and I have shown that asymmetries of the sylvian fissures exist in the great apes but not in monkeys. (Grace H. Yeni-Komshian and Dennis A. Benson have reported similar findings.) If a functional correlative to this anatomical bias can be discovered, an animal model of cerebral dominance in the anthropoid apes would become available.

One of the most commonplace manifestations of cerebral dominance is also one of the most puzzling: the phenomenon of handedness. Many animals exhibit a form of handedness; for example, if a monkey is made to carry out a task with only one hand, it will consistently use the same one. In any large population of monkeys, however, left- and right-handed individuals are equally common. In the human population no more than 9 percent are left-handed. This considerable bias toward right-handedness may represent a unique specialization of the human brain.

The genetics and heritability of handedness is a controversial topic. In mice Robert V. Collins, working at the Jackson Laboratory in Bar Harbor, Me., has shown that continued inbreeding of right-handed animals does not increase the prevalence of right-handedness in their offspring. The pattern in man is quite different. Marian Annett of the Coventry Polytechnic in England has proposed a theory in which one allele of a gene pair favors the development of right-handedness, but there is no complementary allele for left-handedness. In the absence of the right-favoring allele handedness is randomly determined.

Studies undertaken by LeMay and her co-workers have revealed that the distribution of brain asymmetries in left-handed people is different from that in right-handers. In right-handed individuals, and hence in most of the population, the right sylvian fissure is higher than the left in 67 percent of the brains examined. The left fissure is higher in 8 percent and the two fissures rise to approximately equal height in 25 percent. In the left-handed population a substantial majority (71 percent) have approximate symmetry of the sylvian fissures. Among the remainder the right fissure is still more likely to be the higher (21 percent v. 7 percent). The asymmetries observed by tomography also have a different distribution in right-handers and left-handers.

Again in the left-handed segment of the population the asymmetries tend to be less pronounced. These findings are in qualitative agreement with the theory proposed by Annett.

If functions as narrowly defined as facial recognition are accorded specific neural networks in the brain, it seems likely that many other functions are represented in a similar way. For example, one of the major goals of child rearing is to teach a set of highly differentiated responses to emotional stimuli, such as anger and fear. The child must also be taught the appropriate responses to stimuli from its internal milieu, such as hunger or fullness of the bladder or bowel. Most children learn these patterns of behavior just as they learn a language, suggesting that here too special-purpose processors may be present. As yet little is known about such neural systems. Indeed, even as the mapping of specialized regions continues, the next major task must be confronted: that of describing their internal operation.

Turning Something Over in the Mind

The imagined rotation of an object mirrors a physical rotation. The mental process can be investigated objectively, yielding quantitative information about one form of spatial thinking.

· · ·

Lynn A. Cooper and Roger N. Shepard
December, 1984

What is thinking? Introspection supplies preliminary answers. Some thought is verbal: a kind of silent talking to oneself. Other mental processes seem to be visual: images are called to mind and wordlessly manipulated. Evident though they are, the mechanisms of thought long eluded experimental analysis and quantification. How can these seemingly inaccessible, subjective processes be measured and investigated scientifically?

We have begun to provide an answer to this question by devising experiments to probe the nature of one mode of thinking: imagined spatial operations. Our results confirm empirically what is subjectively apparent: that the mind can model physical processes, subjecting them to the geometric constraints that hold in the external world. Evidence of such mental operations abounds in everyday life. Consider this question: How do you take a card table through a narrow doorway without folding up its legs? Most people report that they must envision the process of turning the table on its side, putting two of the legs into the opening, then turning and moving the table so that the legs, the top and the other pair of legs pass through the door.

This kind of spatial imagination may not be peculiar to human beings. One of us witnessed a German shepherd retrieving a long stick that had been thrown over a fence from which one vertical board was missing. The dog bounded through the gap, seized the stick in its mouth and plunged headlong back toward the narrow opening. Just as catastrophe seemed imminent, the dog stopped short, paused and rotated its head 90 degrees. With the stick held vertically it passed through the fence without mishap. The operation that took place in the mind of the dog in the moment before it turned its head presumably was not verbal. Might it not have been a preparatory mental rotation of the stick? (And was it not by spatial visualization rather than verbal deduction that you, the reader, understood how catastrophe threatened and was averted?)

The ability to represent objects or arrangements of objects and their transformations in space clearly is valuable in managing the concrete realities of everyday life, making it possible to plan actions and to anticipate outcomes. It may also play an important role in abstract thought. Many scientists have testified that their greatest achievements grew from imagined spatial relations and transformations. Two well-known cases are Friedrich Kekulé's image of the structure of the benzene molecule and James Watt's visualization of the mechanism of the condensing steam engine. Albert Einstein even remarked that he arrived at the theory of relativity by "visualizing . . . effects, consequences and possibilities" through "more or less clear images which can be 'voluntarily' reproduced and combined."

Yet subjective and qualitative assessments, even those made by scientists, cannot substitute for an objective and quantitative understanding. As the distinguished physiological psychologist K. S. Lashley put it in 1923, "introspection may make the preliminary survey, but it must be followed by the chain and transit of objective measurement." Such systematic inquiry into spatial imagination has been slow in arriving.

For the first half of the 20th century theoretical barriers stood in the way. During this time American behaviorists from J. B. Watson to B. F. Skinner tried to sever psychology from its introspective origins in philosophy and establish it on its own empirical foundations. They insisted that all theoretical terms correspond to objectively specifiable stimuli and responses and banished such references to subjective phenomena as the terms consciousness, mind, thinking and imagining. Laboratory studies focused on physically recordable events such as bar pressing by rats and lever pecking by pigeons rather than on the hidden workings of the mind.

During the second half of the century new developments began to erode the barriers the behaviorists had erected against the study of the structures and processes of thought. The linguist Noam Chomsky made a forceful argument that language behavior is guided by innate schematisms that had gone completely unrecognized by the behaviorists. And experimental psychologists produced increasingly compelling demonstrations that mental processes could be inferred and even quantified from patterns in objectively recorded data.

Our own experiments were designed to probe the kind of mental process the behaviorists ignored in a way that meets the behaviorists' demand for objective and quantitative data. The first of our inquiries into the process of spatial imagination, undertaken in 1971 by one of us (Shepard) with Jacqueline Metzler, a graduate student, met both criteria. Each experimental trial was objective in the sense that the subject's response to a stimulus was either objectively correct or incorrect, and quantitative in the sense that the variable of interest

Figure 8.1 THREE-DIMENSIONAL SHAPES rotated in space are depicted in computer-generated perspective drawings. When the subjects were shown pairs of line drawings portraying the same shape in different orientations, the time they took to recognize that the shapes were identical was proportional to the angular difference in the orientations shown. The linear increase in comparison time with difference in orientation suggested that subjects had to imagine one shape rotated into the orientation of the other in order to check for a match.

was the time it took the subject to respond correctly.

The subjects of the experiment compared computer-generated perspective line drawings presented in pairs. Each drawing portrayed a three-dimensional object composed of 10 cubical blocks joined face to face to form an armlike structure exhibiting three right-angled bends (see Figure 8.1). Certain of the pairs showed identical structures, usually presented in different spatial orientations; others, randomly mixed with the first type in the series of trials, showed structures that differed in both shape and orientation. These pairs portrayed enantiomorphic structures, which differ by a reflection in space, much as a left hand differs from a right.

In each trial the subject looked into a tachistoscope (see Figure 8.2), a darkened box in which visual stimuli placed at the back could be displayed at precisely controlled times. The experimenter inserted a pair of drawings and closed a switch to illuminate them, simultaneously starting a clock. The subject then compared the drawings as quickly as possible and responded by pulling one of two levers: a right-hand lever for pairs that showed the same shape and a left-hand lever for pairs that showed different shapes. Either response stopped the clock, thus recording the time taken for comparison.

Because the pairs of drawings represented objects that either were identical or differed by a reflection in space, subjects could not base their comparison on superficial features of the stimuli. The numbers of blocks between successive bends, for instance, were identical in both drawings whether the structures were identical or enantiomorphic. A short-cut search for obvious differences was ruled out. Subjects reported they could compare the shapes only by imagining one of the two objects rotated into the same orientation as the other and then checking for a match. Typically they said they imagined the object on the left turned until its top arm paralleled the

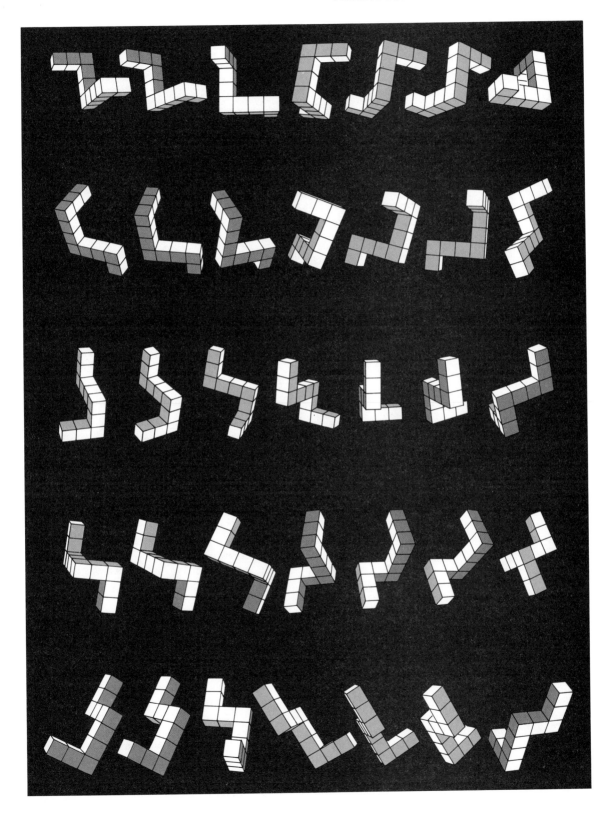

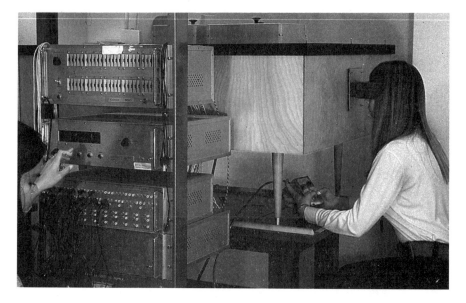

Figure 8.2 TACHISTOSCOPE enables an investigator to time a subject's responses to visual stimuli. When the investigator closes a switch, a display is illuminated, revealing the images, and a timer begins to run. The subject's reaction, registered in the illustrated case through hand-held controls, stops the clock to yield a precise record of the interval between stimulus and response. (Photo by Roger N. Shepard.)

corresponding arm of the right-hand object; they then mentally checked to see whether the extension at the other end of the object projected in the same direction as the analogous section of the companion structure.

The reaction times, measured from the moment the drawings were displayed until each subject responded by pulling a lever, provide objective evidence in support of the subjective accounts. The times increased as a linear function of the angular difference between the orientations portrayed. When like objects were displayed in the same orientation, subjects took about a second to detect identity; with increasing angular difference the response times rose steadily, up to an average of 4.4 seconds for the maximum possible angular difference of 180 degrees. Each of the eight young adults who took part showed a linear increase in reaction time, but the slope of the function varied among individuals (see Figure 8.3).

The linear increases suggest that the subjects compared the objects by imagining one object rotated into the orientation of another at a steady rate that swept out 180 degrees in an average of 3.4 seconds (4.4 minus the second needed to compare two objects in identical orientations), that is, at an average rate of 53 degrees per second. Other methods can be conceived for the discrimination of identical and enantiomorphic objects, but none would take an amount of time proportional to the angular difference. Excluded, for example, is the possibility that subjects analyzed each drawing of a pair separately to reduce its structure to a code of some kind and then compared the coded descriptions. One kind of code might describe the number of blocks and the directions of successive bends, starting at one end of the object: 2R2U2L1 for "two blocks, right bend, two blocks, upward bend, two blocks, left bend, one block," for example. The time needed to generate such a code might depend on the orientation of each object. But because the codes are computed independently, the sum of the times needed to generate codes for two objects need not vary with the angular difference between them.

The results not only point to mental rotation as the basis of this kind of comparison: they also indicate that the subjects' mental images represented the three-dimensional structure of the objects portrayed and not simply the two-dimensional features of the drawings. In half of the same-shape pairs the orientations shown differed by a rotation within the two-dimensional plane of the picture; the two

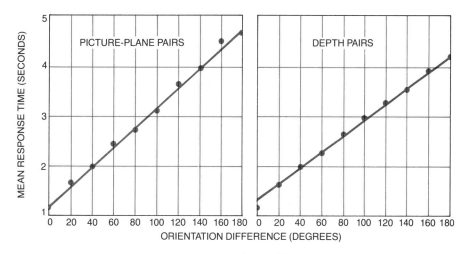

Figure 8.3 MEAN RESPONSE TIMES increased in direct proportion to the angular difference in orientation of identical objects presented for comparison in pairs of drawings. The linear relation suggested that a process of mental rotation underlies such comparisons. The slope of the function, from which the rate of the imagined rotation can be estimated, was no greater for orientations differing by a rotation in depth than for those differing by a rotation in the picture plane.

drawings thus were identical except in position in the plane. The other half of the pairs portrayed objects differing by rotations in depth (see Figure 8.4). Although the three-dimensional objects depicted by each pair of this second set of drawings were identical, the drawings themselves, as two-dimensional arrangements of lines and angles, often differed considerably: a rotation in depth simultaneously shifts some features of a three-dimensional object into the plane of a drawing while removing other features from the picture plane.

Yet the slope of the reaction-time function was no greater for the pairs corresponding to a rotation in depth than it was for those in which the drawings differed by a picture-plane rotation. The rate of imagined rotation was as fast when the transformation portrayed involved three dimensions as it was when the rotation appeared to take place in two dimensions. The results are consistent with subjects' reports that they interpreted all the drawings, whatever the relative orientations, as solid objects in three-dimensional space. The subjects therefore found all rotations equally easy to imagine.

The progressive and spatial nature of imagined rotations, established in the first experiment, suggests that the process is analogous to transformations in the physical world. It is tempting to view the imagined rotation as the internal simulation of an external rotation. Such a description, however, would be justified only if we could demonstrate that the internal process passes through intermediate states corresponding to the intermediate orientations of a physical object rotating in the external world.

To gather this additional evidence for the analogue nature of mental rotation one of us (Cooper) did a series of experiments in which subjects responded not to a pair of objects but to a single figure, displayed at intervals and in a variety of orientations. By triggering an imagined rotation with a single stimulus and then presenting the same or a different object in any orientation and after any delay, we could probe the mental transformation as it was taking place.

Before exploring the ongoing process of rotation, however, an initial question required resolution and therefore a brief experimental digression. We had to establish that the single-stimulus technique causes subjects to imagine the same progressive mental rotations as the paired drawings of the first test did. To evaluate the one-stimulus procedure we again asked subjects to discriminate between an object and its mirror image. In this case we used two-di-

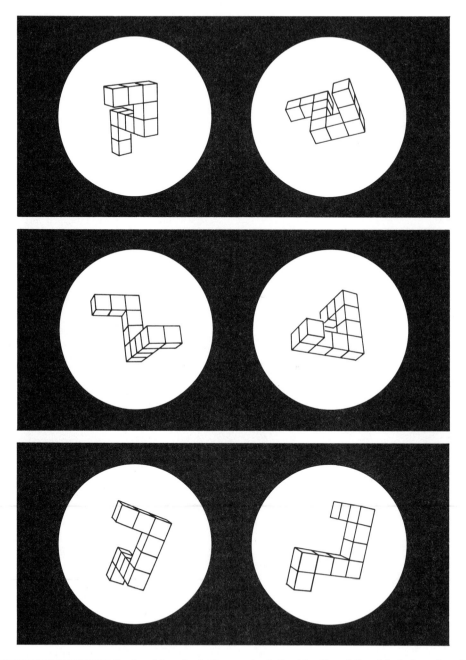

Figure 8.4 PERSPECTIVE VIEWS displayed in pairs to the subjects of the authors' first experiment differed in three ways. In the first case (*top*) the drawings showed identical objects in positions that differed by a rotation within the plane of the picture. In the second (*middle*) the orientations portrayed differed by a rotation in depth. Subjects deter- mined the identity of the objects in pairs of both types equally quickly, which suggests that in both cases they imagined the objects as three-dimensional solids rotating in space in order to compare them. A third kind of drawing pair used in the trials depicted enantiomorphic, or mirror- image, shapes (*bottom*).

mensional plane figures rather than the three-dimensional solids of the earlier experiment. Consequently all the orientations shown differed by rotations in a plane.

The subjects first learned to differentiate standard from mirror-image versions of each of eight polygons, the orientations of which were kept constant throughout this training (see Figure 8.5). Once the subjects had learned the eight discriminations the experimental trials began.

In each trial a subject was shown one of the polygons in an orientation that either matched the training position or differed from it by some multiple of 60 degrees. The subject's task was to determine whether the shape was the standard or the reflected version of the polygon; to make the dis-

crimination the subject presumably had to imagine the polygon rotated until it either matched or did not match the mental representation of the standard shape that had been learned during the training. In the case of a match the subject pressed a right-hand button for "standard"; when there was no match, the subject pressed a left-hand button for "reflected."

Like the paired-stimulus procedure, this test yielded a linear increase in reaction time with increasing angular departure — departure, in this case, from a learned position rather than from the orientation of an object displayed simultaneously. Subjects responded to the standard versions of the test polygons a constant 60 milliseconds faster than they did to the reflected versions; it appeared that sub-

STANDARD VERSIONS   REFLECTED VERSIONS

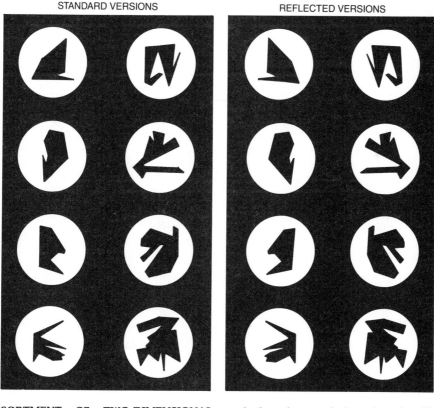

Figure 8.5 ASSORTMENT OF TWO-DIMENSIONAL TEST SHAPES includes eight different polygons and their mirror-image versions. Prior to a set of experiments in which subjects were shown one of the shapes in an unfamiliar orientation each participant learned to discriminate the "standard" (*left*) from the "reflected" (*right*) version of each shape in a particular orientation. The eight shapes vary in the number of points defining their perimeters, a characteristic that may correspond to psychological complexity. Yet the complexity of a shape had no effect on the speed with which subjects later discriminated its standard form from its reflected form.

jects first compared the transformed test shape with a memory of the standard shape and could react to a match immediately but needed an extra interval to initiate the "reflected" response if the shapes did not correspond.

The slopes of the response-time functions for both standard and reflected test shapes were identical, however. The inferred average rate of mental rotation was 450 degrees per second, considerably higher than the 53 degrees per second estimated in the earlier two-stimulus experiment. Evidently the use of plane images presented one at a time allowed swifter responses by enabling subjects to focus their attention on a single stimulus. In spite of quantitative differences the results of this procedure parallel those of the earlier one (see Figure 8.6).

Having determined that the one-stimulus, two-dimensional test requires a mental rotation like that required by the two-stimulus comparison, we could modify the procedure to scrutinize more closely the

hypothesis that mental rotation is analogous to rotations in the physical world. The second of the single-stimulus experiments directly tested subjects' statements that they appraised a stimulus by imagining its turning until it matched the learned shape. In effect we reversed the earlier sequence of events: instead of presenting subjects with a stimulus for comparison with a learned shape, thus requiring them to imagine a corrective rotation, we first asked them to imagine the rotation of a learned shape and only then presented a stimulus for comparison.

All the subjects in this experiment had taken part in the earlier one-stimulus experiment and were familiar with the test shapes. In each trial a subject viewed an outline drawing of one of the eight standard polygons that was displayed in the training orientation. The outline was followed by a circle containing a pointer positioned in one of six equally spaced angular increments from zero de-

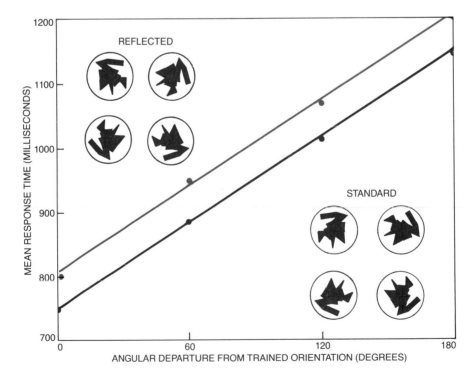

Figure 8.6 LINEAR RELATION OF RESPONSE TIME TO TEST ORIENTATION was found when subjects viewed a familiar polygon in a new orientation and determined whether it was the standard version (*lower graph*) or the reflected version (*upper graph*) of the shape. To evaluate the test shape subjects apparently had to imagine a rotation of the standard shape until it either matched or did not match the shape displayed. If there was no match, it took subjects a consistent extra increment of time to indicate that the shape before them was the reflected version.

grees to 300 degrees of clockwise rotation. The subject then imagined the outlined shape rotated into the orientation indicated by the pointer. In half of the trials the subjects had been instructed to do a clockwise mental rotation; in the other half they had been told to imagine the displayed shape rotated in a counterclockwise direction.

To indicate that the mental operation was complete the subject pressed a button, thus stopping the clock that recorded preparation time. Simultaneously a version of the outlined polygon appeared in the orientation indicated by the arrow and a second clock started. As quickly as possible the subject announced whether the drawing showed the standard or the reflected version of the shape by saying "S" (for "standard") or "R" (for "reflected") into a microphone. A voice-activated relay then stopped the second clock.

Each trial hence yielded two times: the time required to effect the mental rotation and the interval then necessary for the subject to classify a test stimulus. Both sets of results confirmed earlier findings. The time needed for the preparatory mental rotation increased linearly with the angular departure from the training orientation, as earlier results had led us to expect (see Figure 8.7). Moreover, in previous experiments the direction of mental rotation was not specified and the greatest testable rotation was 180 degrees. Here the linear increase in preparation time extended to the maximum clockwise or counterclockwise rotation of 300 degrees, providing further evidence that the mental operation was analogous to a physical rotation. The inferred rate of the preparatory rotations, an average of about 370 degrees per second, was comparable to the 450 degrees per second estimated from the earlier one-stimulus experiment.

The second set of times, which recorded the interval required for subjects to respond to the test stimulus appearing after they signaled readiness, confirmed that the act of mental rotation did in fact prepare them to make the discrimination. On the average they classified each test shape as standard or reflected in less than half a second, regardless of its angular departure from the learned position. If the subjects had needed to do further mental operations after they confronted the test stimulus, response times presumably would have increased with the angular departure of the test stimulus, as they had done in earlier experiments where there was no opportunity for a preparatory mental rotation.

The experiments described so far all document characteristics of completed mental rotations. We found that the time required increases in direct proportion to the angle of rotation, and we confirmed that having imagined a shape rotated into the orientation of a physical stimulus, a subject can determine identity or difference with uniform speed, whatever the degree of rotation. But to characterize the mental process as analogous to physical rotations we still had to show that the mental process passes through stages corresponding to the intermediate angles of a physical rotation. If such a correspondence does exist, the angle at which a displayed shape will elicit the quickest response from an individual who is imagining an ongoing rotation of the shape should change steadily and progressively with time, in step with the mental rotation.

The subjects of a further experiment, designed to test that hypothesis, were all veterans of the two earlier single-stimulus experiments and were familiar with the eight test polygons. On each trial a blank circular field appeared in the tachistoscope and the subject was asked to imagine a specified polygon rotating within the field at the subject's natural rate. After an unpredictable interval that shape or its mirror image appeared; the subject then identified the version as quickly as possible.

Because we already had extensive data on each individual's rate of rotation, we could tailor the trials to the individual subjects. From the earlier experiments we inferred the times and angles at which each subject should be most ready to respond to a test shape. In half of the trials, called the probe-expected trials, the test shape was presented at an angle and time intended to match precisely the ongoing mental rotation. In the other trials the shape was displayed in an orientation that differed by varying angles from what was calculated to be the orientation imagined at that moment. We termed this second kind of trial probe-unexpected.

If a subject necessarily imagines an object in intermediate orientations in the course of mental rotation, the response to a properly timed and oriented probe should be uniformly fast whatever the angle tested is. The reaction times in the probe-expected trials were consistent with our hypothesis: the response times for trials in which the probe was displayed in an expected orientation were virtually constant at about half a second for every angle. (see Figure 8.8, left).

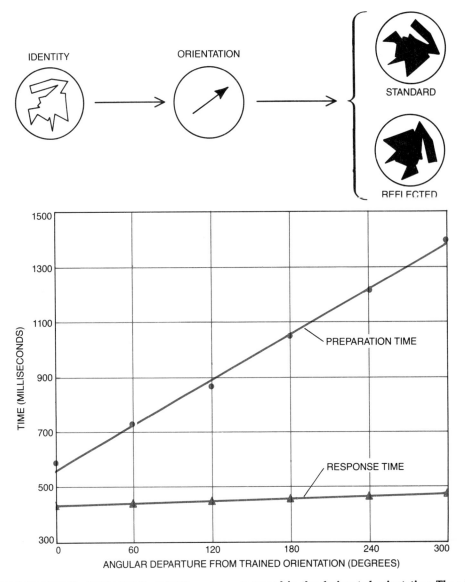

Figure 8.7 PREPARATORY ROTATION TIMES were measured in the experiment shown schematically at the top. Subjects first viewed an outline drawing of one of the eight polygons, followed by an arrow. They imagined the shape, now present only in their memory, rotated into the orientation indicated by the arrow. When the mental operation was complete, they signaled, and a test shape appeared in the designated orientation. They then determined whether the shape was a standard or a reflected version. The time required for the preparatory mental rotation increased linearly with the angle; the consistently fast response to the test shape confirmed that the process of mental rotation prepared subjects to judge the reoriented shape.

Another feature of the probe-expected trials is instructive. The orientations of half of the probes were multiples of 60 degrees—the same orientations that were used in the earlier one-stimulus experiment. The other "expected" probes were dis-played at unfamiliar angles, all odd multiples of 30 degrees. If, as we propose, mental rotation does not jump discontinuously from angle to angle but instead progresses steadily through states corresponding to intermediate angles, the response times to

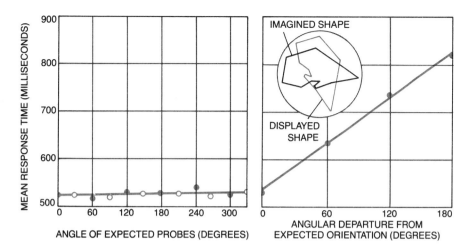

Figure 8.8 PROBING ONGOING MENTAL ROTATIONS. When a subject imagined a shape rotating and the presentation of a test shape was timed so that its orientation matched the momentary orientation of the imagined shape, response times were consistently fast at every angle probed (*left*). The results were not affected by the fact that some of the probes (*open dots*) depicted orientations the subjects had not seen in earlier experiments. When the investigators deliberately mismatched the probe and the orientation the subject was imagining (*right*), response times increased with the angular discrepancy. Subjects presumably had to imagine a compensatory rotation to evaluate the test shape.

properly timed probes in the unfamiliar angles should approximate those for probe angles in which the subjects were well versed. Nearly identical response times at familiar and unfamiliar orientations bore out the hypothesis.

When the probe deviated from the expected orientation, reaction times increased linearly with the angle of the discrepancy (see Figure 8.8, right). Clearly subjects had to imagine a further, correctional rotation when they were presented with a test shape that did not match their current mental representation; the correction took time proportional to the angle of the deviation. The finding provides additional evidence that a correspondence between the imagined and the displayed orientations, and not the subjects' familiarity with the shapes in all orientations, was crucial to the short and constant response times. The correction times indicate that, although the test subjects were practiced, they could not evaluate the displayed shapes without first doing a mental rotation.

Taken together, our results amount to objective evidence of a mental process that models the rotation of objects in the physical world. The two central findings are the linear relation of reaction time to orientation difference when two stimuli are compared for intrinsic shape, and the uniform ra-

pidity of response when a test object is presented in a position calculated to match the steadily changing orientation that is imagined in a mental rotation. We have gathered precise and reproducible data on a seemingly subjective phenomenon of the kind that in the past was considered to lie outside the proper scope of experimental psychology.

Questions still remain about the nature of the mental transformations we have studied. Although we have established that determining the identity of objects displayed in differeing orientations can require imagining a rotation through intermediate orientations, we do not contend that the rotation is continuous in the strict mathematical sense, which requires that it sweep through all possible intermediate angles. The neurophysiological basis of the mental images and of their internal manipulation is not known.

Still other questions remain: How much detail from corresponding physical objects do the mental images preserve as they are transformed? Recent experiments suggest that mental representations can preserve much of the structural richness of their material counterparts. In research conducted by Cooper and Peter Podgorny (a former student) subjects were able to discriminate rotated test shapes from standard shapes not only when the probes differed by reflections in space but also when the

STANDARD
SHAPES

DISTORTIONS

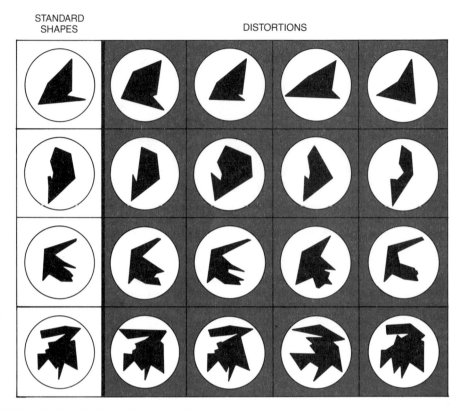

Figure 8.9 DISTORTIONS OF THE STANDARD SHAPES tested the fidelity with which the features of a physical stimulus are retained when it is rotated mentally. After indicating an orientation into which the subjects were to imagine one of the standard shapes as having rotated, the experimenters presented the reoriented standard shape or one of various distortions of it. Subjects could detect even minor variations from the standard shape, which suggests that in the process of mental rotation much of the structural richness of the original shape is preserved.

distinction was a matter of subtle, unpredictable local perturbations (see Figure 8.9).

In spite of some unresolved issues, the close match we have found between mental rotations and their counterparts in the physical world leads inevitably to speculations about the functions and origin of human spatial imagination. It may not be premature to propose that spatial imagination has evolved as a reflection of the physics and geometry of the external world. The rules that govern structures and motions in the physical world may, over evolutionary history, have been incorporated into human perceptual machinery, giving rise to demonstrable correspondences between mental imagery and its physical analogues. We begin to discern here a mental mechanics as precise and elegant as the innate schematism posited by Chomsky as the foundation of language.

A Window on the Sleeping Brain

REM (rapid eye movement) sleep, the phase of sleep when vivid dreams occur, is normally accompanied by paralysis. The paralysis can now be turned off in animals, making it possible to explore the REM phase.

• • •

Adrian R. Morrison
April, 1983

Sleep is ordinarily regarded as a condition of complete relaxation and inactivity. When the electrical activity of the brain in a sleeping human being or experimental animal is observed, however, it becomes evident that sleep is a complex and by no means inactive state. Indeed, the electrical activity of the brain in the phase of sleep when vivid dreams occur—REM (rapid eye movement) sleep—resembles that of wakefulness more closely than it does that of the other phases of sleep. In REM sleep transitory voltage changes indicate that the brain is in a state of arousal, in spite of the fact that sensory contact between the animal and its environment is much reduced. What prevents the neural arousal of the brain in REM sleep from being translated into vigorous physical movement is the absence of activity in the animal's muscles, which results in a paralysis that lasts until an episode of REM sleep ends.

What would happen if the paralysis that accompanies REM sleep were eliminated and the aroused brain were enabled to activate the muscles? Work in my laboratory at the University of Pennsylvania and in other laboratories is beginning to answer the question. The most primitive part of the brain is the brain stem, which lies between the spinal cord and the rest of the brain. In the cat small, precisely controlled lesions in the brain stem result in animals that show the electrical characteristics of REM sleep but move vigorously. The lesions are made in the region of the brain stem called the pons, and the exact position of the lesion within the pons strongly affects which muscles are freed from paralysis (see Figure 9.1).

Therefore the lack of muscle tone in sleep appears to be directly attributable to the pons. Other experimental results suggest that neurons (nerve cells) in the pons also affect locomotion indirectly. In REM sleep one region of the pons appears to interfere with the action of a "locomotion center" that extends from the pons to a point farther down the brain stem. This interference prevents the locomotion center from activating the nerve networks in the spinal cord that are responsible for the reciprocal (alternating) motion of the limbs. Thus the activity of the pons in REM sleep leads to the inhibition of movement in two ways. My own work suggests that the link between heightened brain activity and muscular paralysis can also operate in wakefulness and may be the cause of certain sleep disorders.

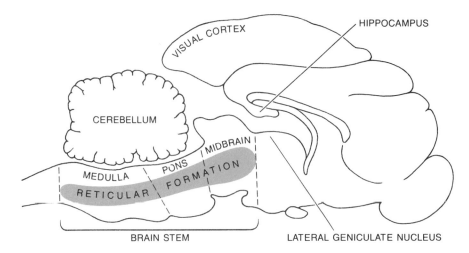

Figure 9.1 BRAIN STRUCTURES that play a role in sleep are indicated in a schematic section of the brain of a cat. The front of the brain is to the right. The lesions that eliminate paralysis in REM sleep are in the pons, a structure in the brain stem between the medulla and the midbrain.

The transition from alert wakefulness to sleep entails many changes in an animal's physiology and posture; the alterations collectively result in a profound change of state. Much of my work has been done with cats, and the changes described here apply specifically to the cat, but many of them are shared by other mammalian species. When a cat falls asleep, it assumes a familiar curled-up and relaxed pose. Its eyes close, and the nictitating membrane (the "third eyelid") covers part of the eye under the outer eyelids. There is a reduction in the number of muscle fibers that are contracting and therefore a reduction in the degree of tone in the muscles. In the initial phase of sleep the movements of the eye that can be detected in the waking animal disappear. There is a gradual lowering of brain temperature, generally by a fraction of a degree Celsius.

Underlying such changes are the changes in the neural activity of the brain that occur when sleep begins. The most general information about the electrical activity of the brain is provided by the electroencephalogram (EEG). The EEG is a record of continuous changes in electric potential measured between electrodes affixed to the skull. The rapid changes in potential represent the sum of changes in voltage in the outer membrane of large numbers of brain neurons.

The EEG in an awake and alert cat shows waves with a relatively low amplitude and a relatively high frequency. As the cat curls up and goes to sleep, there is a notable change (see Figure 9.2). The low-amplitude waves of wakefulness are replaced gradually by high-amplitude, low-frequency waves. Because of the presence of the low-frequency pattern in the EEG, the light initial phase of sleep is often referred to as slow-wave sleep. As the animal enters slow-wave sleep, there are also changes in electrical activity in specific areas of the upper and lower brain. Such changes are recorded by means of electrodes inserted into the appropriate brain structure.

For many years the slow-wave pattern was thought to prevail throughout sleep. In 1953, however, Eugene Aserinsky and Nathaniel Kleitman, working at the University of Chicago, noted in human beings intervals of sleep when the EEG record reverted to the high-frequency, low-amplitude pattern of wakefulness. After the EEG pattern had changed, the sleepers' eyes were periodically observed to move rapidly in various directions; it is for this reason that the intervals have been designated rapid-eye-movement sleep. Periods of REM sleep are now known to recur regularly during sleep, alternating with longer periods of slow-wave sleep. The timing and the duration of the REM periods vary with the species. REM sleep comes about once every 90 minutes in human beings and about once every 25 minutes in cats. Each episode lasts for several minutes.

By waking sleepers immediately after an episode

of rapid eye movement had ended Aserinsky and Kleitman were able to show that REM sleep is associated with vivid and intense dreams. The identification of the time in sleep when the sleeper dreams was the source of much of the initial excitement over the discovery of REM sleep. Later work has shown, however, that the physiological aspects of REM sleep are equally intriguing.

In addition to the essentially identical EEG patterns in REM sleep and in the waking state the rates of activity of neurons in most of the subunits of the brain are quite similar in the two states. One of the most striking similarities is found in the hippocampus, which is phylogenetically the oldest part of the cerebral cortex. Throughout much of both REM sleep and wakefulness there is a regular pattern of waves in the hippocampus at a rate of about seven per second. This pattern, the "theta rhythm," is quite different from the activity of the hippocampus in slow-wave sleep, which is less regular and shows spike-like waves. An additional similarity is in brain temperature: after decreasing part of a degree in slow-wave sleep, the temperature of the brain increases to roughly the waking level during an episode of REM sleep.

Hence many of the characteristics of REM sleep are parallel to those of wakefulness and are quite different from the characteristics of slow-wave sleep. Remarkably, all the characteristics mentioned above are signs of activation of the reticular formation, or reticular activating system, in the core of the brain stem. In 1949 Giuseppe Moruzzi and Horace W. Magoun, working together at Northwestern University, demonstrated that the reticular formation is responsible for arousal. Thus in REM sleep the brain is highly aroused. Because of the juxtaposition of rest and arousal, REM sleep is sometimes called paradoxical sleep.

The close connection between REM sleep and alert wakefulness was emphasized recently by an unexpected finding in my laboratory. One of my students, Robert Bowker, had been working on electrical waves in REM sleep that appear "spontaneously" (meaning without apparent external stimulation). These brief, high-amplitude waves are called PGO spikes in reference to the brain structures in which they have been most studied: the pons (where they are thought to originate) and two parts of the visual system, the lateral geniculate body and the visual cortex (the occipital region of the cerebral cortex).

It had been thought that PGO spikes were limited almost exclusively to REM sleep and occurred only rarely in slow-wave sleep. One day in the laboratory, however, Bowker accidentally tapped on the recording cage while a record was being made from the brain of a cat in slow-wave sleep. Almost immediately a PGO spike appeared in the record. Further work showed that PGO spikes could be readily elicited in either REM sleep or slow-wave sleep by sounds and by tactile stimuli. Hence PGO spikes, which were thought to be spontaneous electrical events occurring only in REM sleep, were seen to be multisensory alerting responses that can be evoked in several brain states.

The conclusion that PGO spikes are alerting responses led Bowker to reexamine the waves called eye-movement potentials (EMP) that appear in the waking state (see Figure 9.3, top). Such waves in the electrical record are identical in appearance with PGO spikes and are observed in the same brain structures (see Figure 9.3, bottom). The presence of eye-movement potentials, however, was thought to depend on the level of illumination in the cat's environment. Such potentials had not been observed in awake cats in the dark. The dependence of eye-movement potentials on illumination was thought to constitute a significant difference from PGO spikes.

Reasoning that a cat in a dark recording chamber might be somewhat bored, Bowker aroused the animals' interest by sending the odor of tuna fish wafting through the cage. Soon the cat's record showed eye-movement potentials that were identical with PGO spikes. Short bursts of a loud tone yielded the same result. The result suggests that both PGO spikes and eye-movement potentials are particular forms of a general alerting response. The response can be elicited by stimulation in the waking state, in slow-wave sleep or in REM sleep. Activation of the same neurons can apparently also occur spontaneously in REM sleep. Thus in an episode of REM sleep the brain is aroused to the extent that it is in a state resembling alert wakefulness even though sensory contact with the environment is greatly reduced.

What prevents the animal in REM sleep, whose central nervous system is aroused and alert but for the most part cut off from sensory contact with the world, from injuring itself? The answer is that in each period of REM sleep the action of the motor neurons of the spinal cord that cause the skeletal (voluntary) muscles to contract is inhibited. As a

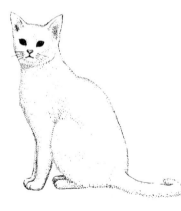

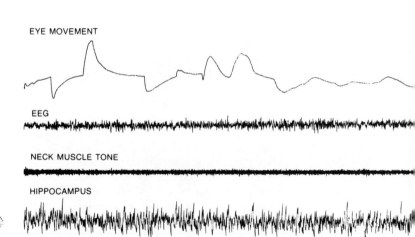

EYE MOVEMENT

EEG

NECK MUSCLE TONE

HIPPOCAMPUS

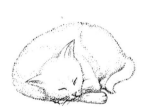

EYE MOVEMENT

EEG

NECK MUSCLE TONE

HIPPOCAMPUS

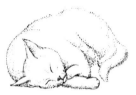

EYE MOVEMENT

EEG

NECK MUSCLE TONE

HIPPOCAMPUS

Figure 9.2 DURING WAKEFULNESS in the cat (*top*) the animal's eyes and head move as the animal responds to visual and auditory stimuli. The electroencephalogram (EEG) shows a pattern of low-amplitude, high-frequency waves. There is substantial tone in the skeletal (voluntary) muscles. The hippocampus shows a regular pattern called the theta rhythm when the cat is attentive to an object. As the animal enters slow-wave sleep (*middle*), it curls up. Eye movements cease. The EEG shows a low-frequency, high-amplitude pattern. Muscle tone decreases and the hippocampus shows an irregular rhythm. When the animal enters REM sleep (*bottom*), the curled-up posture relaxes slightly. Rapid eye movements, a high-frequency EEG pattern and the theta rhythm reappear. Skeletal muscle tone, however, disappears completely, a condition that is referred to as atonia.

the maintenance of upright posture. As we have seen, when the cat enters light sleep, the tone in its muscles decreases because there is a decrease in the number of active fibers in each muscle. When the animal enters a period of REM sleep, the record of muscle tone goes flat, indicating a complete lack of tone. There are occasional bursts of muscle activity, however, that result in twitches in various parts of the body. In my laboratory we have been working with cats in which the atonia of REM sleep has been reversed by means of lesions in the pons made by destroying a small volume of tissue with a heated wire. The wire is introduced into the brain at predetermined coordinates.

After such a lesion is made, remarkable activity is sometimes observed. The activity follows a period of slow-wave sleep, at the time when the cat would ordinarily enter REM sleep with atonia. The cats raise their head, right their body and exhibit alternating movements of their limbs. They attempt to stand, and some succeed; others are actually able to walk. Cats with certain lesions display other behavior usually seen in wakefulness. They make motions typical of orienting toward prey, searching for prey and attacking. These movements are rarely directed at anything in the environment (see Figure 9.4).

result the muscles are atonic, or without tone, and the animal is paralyzed. (It should be noted that atonia and paralysis are not identical. Paralysis can be the result of several conditions other than atonia. If the muscles are atonic, however, the animal will necessarily be paralyzed.)

The degree of activity in the skeletal muscles is often recorded by means of an electrode inserted into the neck. The neck muscles are among the "antigravity" muscles that are responsible for

As I have noted, the kind of muscular activity the

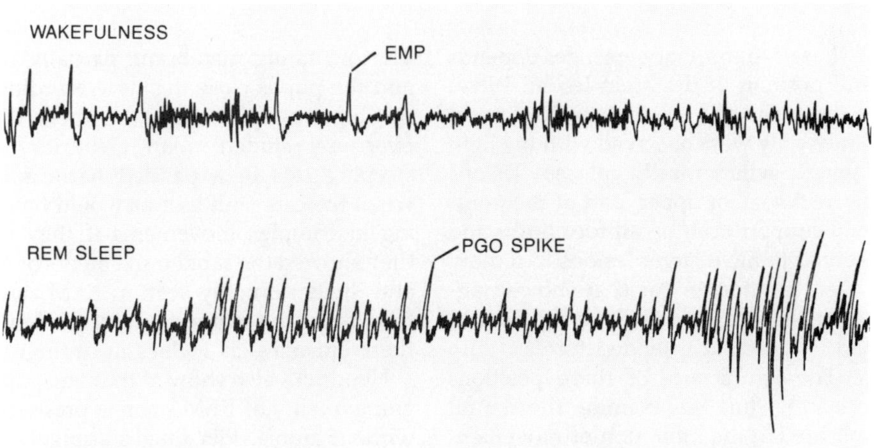

Figure 9.3 BRAIN AROUSAL IN REM SLEEP. In the waking state eye-movement potentials (EMP) appear in the visual area of the cerebral cortex (*top*). Such potentials had been thought to depend solely on the level of illumination. Robert Bowker showed that eye-movement potentials can be elicited by a variety of stimuli even in absolute darkness: they are multisensory alerting responses. Such waves are identical with the waves known as PGO spikes that appear spontaneously in the same areas of the brain in REM sleep (*bottom*). In REM sleep the brain is alert, which results from the brain's activity rather than from sensory information.

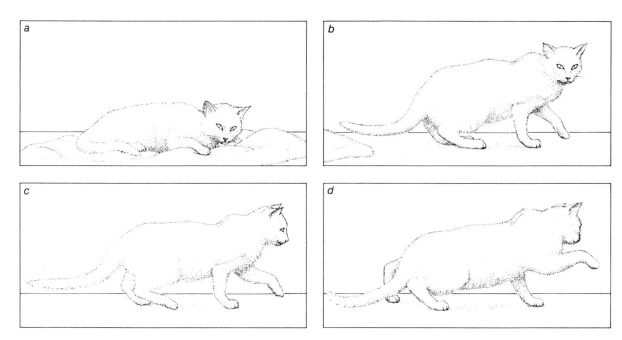

Figure 9.4 REM SLEEP WITHOUT PARALYSIS is shown in drawings based on motion pictures of a cat made in the author's laboratory. The paralysis that normally accompanies REM sleep is eliminated by making a small lesion in the brain stem of the cat; the degree to which the paralysis is eliminated varies with the lesion. The cat in the filmed episode raised its head and righted itself during REM sleep (a). It managed to stand (b) and began to walk (c). It then began to paw at the air in a corner of the laboratory (d). In such episodes the cat shows all the signs of normal REM sleep, including the extension of the nictitating membrane to cover much of the eye. That not all the muscle tone is released is suggested by the cat's slightly swaybacked appearance.

cat displays in these extraordinary episodes depends on the size and position of the brain lesion. When sections from the brain of a cat that could support itself on forelimbs only were observed with the light microscope, small symmetrically placed lesions were noted in the dorsal, or upper, part of the pons. A cat that could support itself on all four limbs and walk was observed to have larger lesions in a more ventral, or lower, position. A cat that showed aggressive behavior, striking repeatedly at the floor in front of it, had lesions that extended forward into the midbrain. The significance of these positions will become clearer when we examine the neural pathways implicated in the inhibition of movement during REM sleep.

Several items of information suggest that the unusual movements we observe do indeed constitute REM sleep without atonia. The phenomenon was initially recognized by Michel Jouvet and François Delorme at the University of Lyons. As in ordinary REM sleep, the EEG of the cats that are active in sleep resembles that of wakefulness (see Figure 9.5).

The nictitating membrane partially covers the eye and the pupils close to slits. Recordings made from the hippocampus show the theta rhythm. Moreover, my student Joan Hendricks confined the sleeping cats in a padded harness, and at times when the cats with lesions would have been engaging in complex movements if they had been free they showed the rapid movements of eyes, whiskers and digits normally seen in REM sleep. Hendricks found that the temperature of the brain rose during these episodes, as it does in ordinary REM sleep.

Hendricks also showed that one particularly intriguing quality of REM sleep is present in REM sleep without atonia. Pier Luigi Parmiggiani and his colleagues at the University of Bologna demonstrated that the capacity of the cat to regulate its body temperature is suspended in REM sleep. In REM sleep cats appear to be "cold-blooded," like fishes, amphibians and reptiles. Hendricks showed that in REM sleep without atonia cats do not shiver or fluff up their coat in response to cold, although the same animals do show such responses when they are

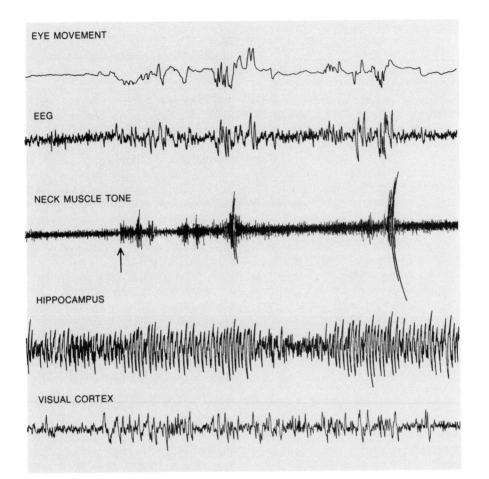

EYE MOVEMENT

EEG

NECK MUSCLE TONE

HIPPOCAMPUS

VISUAL CORTEX

Figure 9.5 EPISODES OF MOVEMENT DURING SLEEP in the cats with lesions take place when all signs except muscle tone are similar to those of REM sleep. It has been concluded that the episodes of movement represent REM sleep without atonia. Recordings from normal REM sleep include rapid eye movement, low-amplitude EEG pattern, theta rhythm and PGO spikes. All are present in record-ings made during the episodes with movement that follow damage to the pons. The notable difference is that in REM sleep without atonia the cat's skeletal muscles have re-gained much tone, enabling the animal to move. Arrow indicates the start of an episode of movement during REM sleep.

awake. Thus the lesions in the pons do not restore the capacity to respond to cold.

Much of my current work is aimed at under-standing how the small lesions in the pons cause the atonia of REM sleep to be reversed and lead to elaborate movements that appear to be much like those of a waking animal. We have con-centrated on the pons because in 1962, early in his work on sleep, Jouvet demonstrated that cats de-prived of the entire brain in front of the pons still showed periods of atonia and rapid eye movements that were identical with those of REM sleep. In the

course of my work I have concluded that there are at least two separate neural systems operating in REM sleep without atonia. One system is responsi-ble for the release of muscle tone, the other for the liberation of "motor drive," a generalized impulse toward locomotion.

The first system appears to be the simpler of the two. It is known that an inhibitory center in the medulla is operative in REM sleep. (The action of neurons can be either excitatory or inhibitory. In-hibitory areas reduce the excitability of the target neurons.) In REM sleep the inhibitory center in the medulla interferes with the spinal neurons that activate the skeletal muscles. This mechanism is thought to be responsible for the lack of tone in the skeletal muscles.

If the inhibitory center in the medulla were in turn under the excitatory control of a network of nerve cells in the pons, damage to the pons could break the excitatory connection. The action of the inhibitory center in the medulla would be interrupted and the skeletal muscles would retain their tone in REM sleep. The extent of the release of tone, and hence the muscles the cats could employ, would depend on the position of the lesions.

This hypothesis has received support from results obtained by Jouvet and his colleagues at Lyons. They have shown that a tract of nerve fibers originates in an area just dorsal to the area in the pons where we made lesions. The tract leads directly to the inhibitory area in the medulla. We have made lesions in the origin and in the course of the tract. Such damage yields cats that have some neck muscle tone in REM sleep but can lift their head only a little. This suggests that other neurons, probably in the reticular formation, must be damaged to release muscle tone completely.

Therefore some experimental evidence bears out the notion that a fairly direct connection between the pons, the inhibitory center in the medulla and the skeletal muscles underlies the atonia of REM sleep. Since REM sleep in human beings is known to be associated with intense dreams, it would be tempting to conclude that by breaking this connection we are enabled to witness the animal acting out its dreams. Apart from the difficulties inherent in attributing complex mental states to other species, however, there are good reasons to think this is not a full account of what happens in the episodes of REM sleep without atonia.

The functions of the brain are carried out by closely interconnected anatomical structures. It would be unreasonable to expect that the only result of damaging a central area of the brain stem would be to destroy structures inhibiting motor neurons. Indeed, we have evidence that systems other than the inhibitory one in the medulla are affected by the lesions in the pons.

The most important evidence concerns the overall level of locomotor activity when the cats with lesions are awake. The cats show no abnormal increase in muscle tone in slow-wave sleep or in wakefulness; the only effect on muscle tone is in REM sleep. Nevertheless, the cats appear to be more active in general than they were before the lesions were made. When they are loose in the laboratory, they make something of a nuisance of themselves, running here and there to investigate inconsequential things.

In order to confirm the impression of unusual locomotor activity we conducted open-field tests. Several cats were tested before and after the lesions were made. The cats were put in a room with a floor that had been marked off in squares. The number of squares each cat entered in a 30-minute period served as a measure of locomotor activity. All the cats that displayed REM sleep without atonia also demonstrated increased activity after the lesions. The increases ranged from 30 to 261 percent and were all significant in a statistical sense. This finding led me to conclude that the lesions in the pons affect a source of generalized motor drive. It is probably an anatomical system different from the one that affects muscle tone, since when the animals were awake, their muscle tone was not affected by the lesions.

Our work is beginning to yield a picture of how the second system of inhibition in sleep could work. My hypothesis of how the system operates borrows heavily from work done on the neural control of locomotion. It has been shown that the region of the brain stem we are interested in can regulate locomotion without any contribution from higher brain centers. Such regulation involves three structures. A "locomotion generator" in the spine includes neurons that control and coordinate the reciprocal motion of the limbs in walking and running. The generator is under the excitatory control of a second structure: a "locomotion center" in the brain stem. If the locomotion center is stimulated, it in turn stimulates the generator of reciprocal motion. The third structure is a control region in the pons, which is connected to the locomotion center by an inhibitory link. When the control region is activated, it suppresses the activity in the locomotion center. Thus in REM sleep the pons could indirectly suppress motor drive as well as muscle tone. Conversely, damage to the pons could release the muscles utilized in locomotion.

The existence of the brain-stem locomotion center and the spinal movement generator has been postulated by many workers, but their anatomical organization is not yet understood. The first evidence of the existence of the locomotion center was obtained by M. L. Shik, F. V. Severin and G. N. Orlovskii of the Moscow State University; their results have

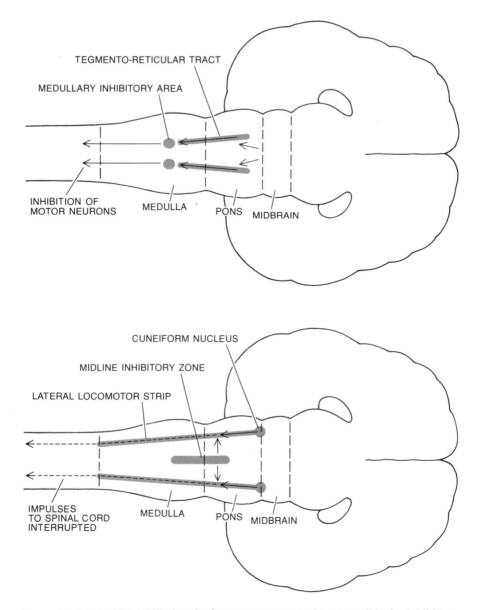

Figure 9.6 SEPARATE NETWORKS of neurons appear to be responsible for inhibiting muscle tone and locomotor drive in REM sleep. An area in the medulla that inhibits motor neurons plays an important role in reducing muscle tone (*upper panel*). The tegmento-reticular tract connects the pons to the inhibitory center. In REM sleep the pons is activated, exciting the medullary center by this pathway and others. The medullary center inhibits the motor neurons and gives rise to atonia. A lateral locomotor strip, down the outside of the brain stem, plays an important part in the reduction of motor drive (*lower panel*). It is connected to structures in the spinal cord and can induce limb motion from which the cerebrum in front of the midbrain has been removed. In REM sleep the pons stimulates the inhibitory zone, turning off the locomotor strip and shutting down motor drive.

since been confirmed by other workers. Shik and his colleagues have shown that the application of an electric current to a neural system originating in the cuneiform nucleus, which is in the caudal region of the midbrain, can cause cats that have been deprived of the cerebrum to walk on a moving treadmill and even to trot or gallop. I suspect it is this center that the lesions in the pons release from inhibition in REM sleep.

Recent work by Shigemi Mori and his coworkers at the Ashikawa Medical College in Japan supports the existence of the locomotion center and suggests how the center may be connected to the pons. The Japanese workers have found that the tracts capable of inducing locomotion in cats deprived of the cerebrum extend from the midbrain down the outer part of the brain stem, in the form of two thin strips passing down the sides of the pons and the medulla. Moreover, they have shown that there are areas in the central part of the brain stem capable of facilitating or inhibiting the operation of the locomotion center (see Figure 9.6).

Whether the locomotion center is excited or inhibited depends on the precise area that is stimulated. Electrical stimulation of the more ventral facilitatory zone is capable of inducing reciprocal movement of the animal's hind legs without any direct stimulation of the locomotion center itself. Dorsal stimulation reduces muscle tone and inhibits locomotion. The facilitatory and inhibitory zones discovered by Mori and his colleagues are near the midline of the brain stem and are close to the regions in the pons where our lesions are made. Thus the connection between the pons and the putative locomotion center is becoming clearer (see Figure 9.7).

Such findings have implications for interpreting the effects of the lesions in the pons. For example, in the cat mentioned above that was able to stand and walk, the lesion was capable of cutting off the full effect of the midline inhibitory zone on the locomotion center. In the cat that could raise itself on its forelimbs only, the lesion was not capable of interrupting the full midline inhibitory effect. My associate Graziella Mann and I have recently found that additional damage to the inhibitory zone in a cat capable of raising itself on forelimbs only can enable the cat to walk on all fours in REM sleep without atonia. Nevertheless, the anatomical connections in the pons and between the locomotion center and the spinal generator remain speculative. Further work in this area is much needed. In the cats that show aggressive behavior there are additional complications. Such animals always have damage in the neural pathways descending from the cerebrum that are known to be involved in the control of aggression in wakefulness.

It should not be assumed, however, that even when the specific anatomical connections have been worked out, the control of the muscles in REM sleep will be completely understood. Even subtler mechanisms than the ones visualized here could be operating. For example, René Drucker-Colin of the University of Mexico and his students Gloria Arankowsky and Raul Aguilar and I have recently shown that the high-frequency neuron discharges occurring in many regions of the brain in REM sleep are necessary for the release of activity in REM sleep without atonia.

The administration of chloramphenicol, a common antibiotic, at a dose comparable to that employed in treating bacterial infection causes atonia to reappear in cats with lesions in the pons that would otherwise show episodes of movement in REM sleep. The cats appear to be normal when they are awake. Drucker-Colin had previously demonstrated that chloramphenicol reduces the rate of firing of the neurons in the reticular formation. The mechanism by which the neural activity is reduced is not known. Chloramphenicol, however, is known to be an inhibitor of protein synthesis, and this action could be responsible for the reeduction in the firing rate of the neurons. Whatever the mechanism of the drug is, after it is administered the lesioned cats appear to have too little locomotor drive to generate the elaborate activity they would otherwise show in REM sleep.

The work that has been done so far on REM sleep without atonia indicates there is a link between the heightened arousal of REM sleep and the reduction of coordinated motor activity. Obviously an organism is well served by a mechanism that makes it impossible to move when the brain is very active but unresponsive to external stimulation. Teleological arguments need not be invoked, however, to explain the existence of a connection between brain arousal and motor inhibition. Such a connection could well exist even in the waking state.

Faced with a novel or unexpected stimulus, a per-

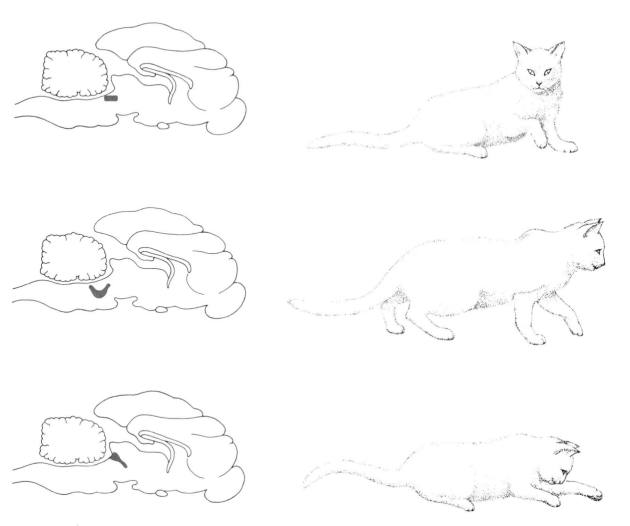

Figure 9.7 POSITION OF LESIONS in the brain of the cat strongly affects the kind of movement the animal shows in REM sleep without atonia. A cat with a small lesion high in the pons could support itself on its forelegs only (*top*). Such a lesion can interrupt only part of the effect of the midline inhibitory zone on the locomotor strip shown in

Figure 9.6. A cat with a larger lesion deeper in the pons stood on all fours and walked (*middle*). Such a lesion can cut off the full effect of the inhibitory zone. A cat with a lesion extending into the midbrain displayed aggressive behavior (*bottom*). Such a lesion affects neural pathways from the cerebrum that regulate aggressive behavior.

son or an animal normally hesitates to some degree before acting. Most people have experienced a moment of hesitation or even a slack feeling in the knees when they have seen a fast-moving automobile bearing down on them. Such waking motor inhibition is generally short-lived. Nevertheless, it suggests that even in wakefulness there is a connection between momentarily heightened alertness and reduced motor activity.

The investigation of this link could have at least

one important clinical consequence. The disorder called narcolepsy is characterized by sudden and unpredictable lapses from wakefulness directly into REM sleep or from wakefulness into paralysis without loss of consciousness. Intriguingly, strong stimulation (such as that accompanying anger, laughter, surprise or sexual intercourse) are the commonest causes of narcoleptic seizure. It is possible that in those who suffer from narcolepsy there is an abnormally low threshold for the link between arousal and motor inhibition; common arousing stimuli could thus lead to atonia or to REM sleep in its entirety at inappropriate moments.

In addition to its possible clinical consequences the investigation of REM sleep without atonia will probably yield further information about the nature of REM sleep itself. It has already helped to clarify one central problem. As we have seen, in most regions of the brain the neurons follow the same pattern in the transition from being awake to being asleep. There is a decrease in the rate of activity from wakefulness to slow-wave sleep and then an increase to the rate of the waking state as an episode of REM sleep begins. Among the neurons that show a different pattern are those of the area of the pons known as the dorsal raphe nucleus. These cells utilize the substance serotonin as a transmitter to alter the activity of the neurons to which they are connected. The rate at which the cells fire decreases from about two impulses per second in wakefulness to almost zero in REM sleep after passing through an intermediate level in slow-wave sleep.

It has been suggested that the inactivity of the neurons in the dorsal raphe nucleus is a fundamental characteristic of REM sleep. Indeed, it had been hypothesized that the decrease in activity causes REM sleep to begin. To test these propositions I collaborated with Barry L. Jacobs and Michael Trulson. Jacobs and Trulson had already thoroughly studied the activity of the dorsal raphe neurons in the waking state and in normal sleep. When we recorded the activity of these cells in REM sleep without atonia, however, the results were surprising. In the cats with lesions in the pons the raphe neurons, instead of falling silent, increased their activity again after slow-wave sleep. The increase was to a rate of about one impulse per second and so did not bring the neurons to the rate in wakefulness. It did, however, yield a rate about six times that of normal REM sleep.

There are at least two plausible explanations for this unexpected finding. The first is that the unusual muscular activity in REM sleep without atonia somehow causes information to be relayed back to the pons to excite the neurons in the dorsal raphe nucleus. An alternative explanation is that the lesions in the pons affect a more central motor mechanism that normally inhibits the raphe neurons in REM sleep. The first hypothesis depends on the relaying of impulses from the periphery of the nervous system to its center whereas the second depends only on events in the brain.

To test the alternative explanations Jacobs and his students employed two drugs. The first is succinylcholine, a drug that is chemically closely related to curare. Succinylcholine acts at the junction between a motor neuron and the muscle cell that the neuron activates. By interrupting the connection the drug induces a temporary paralysis. When succinylcholine was injected into awake normal cats, the raphe neurons remained as active as they had been before the injection. Therefore the raphe neurons could be active in wakefulness with paralysis and in REM sleep without atonia and hence without paralysis. Since the raphe neurons were active in the awake, paralyzed animals, we concluded that the neurons of the raphe nucleus were not being stimulated in REM sleep without atonia by information relayed from the periphery as the result of vigorous muscular activity.

The second drug, carbachol, causes paralysis by directly affecting the mechanism described above that is responsible for atonia. The injection of carbachol silenced the raphe neurons almost completely. Rather than being a fundamental part of REM sleep or even an element in the mechanism that brings on an episode of REM sleep, the inactivity of the dorsal raphe neurons thus appears to be an ancillary phenomenon. It seems to be related to the central motor inhibition of REM sleep, which can be reversed by damage to the pons. Recently my student Peter Reiner has studied the other group of nerve cells that are turned off in REM sleep. These neurons lie near the site of our lesions and employ noradrenaline as a transmitter. Reiner's preliminary results suggest that the inactivity of these cells is also related to the motor inhibition of REM sleep.

By means of experimental techniques that enable us to separate the muscular paralysis associated with deep sleep from the activity that goes on in the brain we are learning much about what is fundamental to REM sleep and what is a side effect of REM-sleep episodes. The current hypotheses concerning the paralysis of REM sleep will undoubtedly require further work to be fully accepted, in particular the notion advanced above of separate pathways for the inhibition of muscle tone and of motor drive and the hypothesis that the second pathway is active in some way in wakefulness.

Whether or not these ideas prove to be sound, REM sleep without atonia will continue to be a

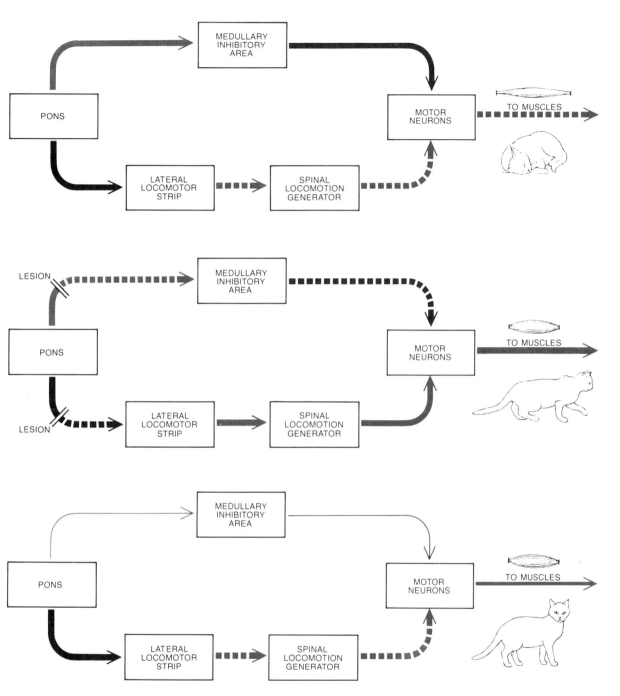

Figure 9.8 SYSTEMS THAT INHIBIT MOVEMENT IN REM SLEEP may also operate in physical emergencies in wakefulness. Excitatory connections are shown in color and inhibitory connections in black. In normal REM sleep the pons strongly activates the inhibitory center in the medulla (*top*). The midline inhibitory zone in the pons inhibits the lateral locomotor strip. The result is complete paralysis. In REM sleep without paralysis the lesions break the connections from the pons to the locomotor strip and to the medullary center (*middle*). The cat can move, but the release of muscle tone is generally not complete. In wakefulness when an unexpected threatening stimulus is perceived, there is sometimes a transitory inhibition of movement (*bottom*). The temporary inhibition is **probably the result of a reduction of motor drive, since there is little loss of muscle tone.**

valuable experimental technique. In addition to making it possible to separate the essential from the ancillary in REM sleep, REM sleep without atonia could provide a means of studying complex behavior such as that of aggression, which is usually elicited in response to external stimuli but which could in REM sleep be generated in isolation from the animal's environment. Furthermore, because of the similarities between wakefulness and REM sleep it will undoubtedly continue to be interesting to compare the two states (see Figure 9.8). In the movements of the waking animal we have a correlate of its inner states. Until now we have lacked such a correlate for REM sleep. In REM sleep without atonia we have acquired a correlate, which is in a sense a window on the sleeping brain.

SECTION

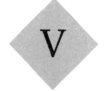

BRAIN MODELS

. . .

Collective Computation in Neuronlike Circuits

Electronic circuits based on neurobiological models are able to solve complex problems rapidly. Their computational properties emerge from the collective interaction of many parts linked together in a network.

. . .

David W. Tank and John J. Hopfield
December, 1987

Modern digital computers are latecomers to the world of computation. Biological computers—the brain and nervous system of animals and human beings—have existed for millions of years, and they are marvelously effective in processing sensory information and controlling the interactions of animals with their environment. Tasks such as reaching for a sandwich, recognizing a face or remembering things associated with the taste of madeleines are computations just as much as multiplication and runnng video games are.

The fact that biological computation is so effective suggests that it may be possible to attain similar capabilities in artificial devices based on the design principles of neural systems. We have studied a number of "neural network" electronic circuits that can carry out significant computations. Such simple models have only a metaphorical resemblance to nature's computers, but they offer an elegant, different way of thinking about machine computation, which is inspiring new microelectronic chip and computer designs. They may also provide fresh insights into the biological systems.

Current research on this subject builds on a long history of efforts to capture the principles of biological computation in mathematical models. The effort began with the pioneering investigations of neurons as logical devices by Warren S. McCulloch and Walter H. Pitts in 1943. In the 1960's Frank Rosenblatt of Cornell University and Bernard Widrow, who is now at Stanford University, created "adaptive neurons" and simple networks that learn. Widrow's Adaline (short for adaptive linear element) is a single-neuron system that can learn to recognize a pattern such as a letter regardless of its orientation or size. Through the 1960's and 1970's a small number of investigators such as Shunichi Amari, Leon N. Cooper, Kunihiko Fukushima and Stephen Grossberg attempted to model the behavior of real neurons in computational networks more closely and to develop mathematics and architectures for extracting features from patterns, for classifying patterns and for "associative memory," in which pieces of the stored information itself serve to retrieve an entire memory.

The 1980's have seen an extraordinary growth of interest in neural models and their computational properties. Many factors converged to bring this about: neurobiologists were gaining more understanding of how information is processed in nature, cheap computer power made it possible to analyze the models in detail and there was growing interest in parallel computation and analog VLSI (very-large-scale integration), which lend themselves to implementations of neuronlike circuits. New concepts in the mathematics of neural models accompanied these developments. Our work has focused on the principles that give rise to computational behavior in a particular type of neuronlike circuit.

Neurons, or nerve cells, are complex, but even a highly simplified model of a neuron, when it is connected with others in an appropriate network, can do significant computations. A biological neuron receives information from other neurons through synaptic connections and passes on signals to as many as a thousand other neurons. The synapse, or connection between neurons, mediates the "strength" with which a signal crosses from one neuron to another. One can readily build artificial "neural" circuits from simple electronic components: operational amplifiers replace the neurons, and wires, resistors and capacitors replace the synaptic connections. The output voltage of the amplifier represents the activity of the model neuron, and currents through the wires and resistors represent the flow of information in the network.

Strikingly, both the simplified biological model and the artificial network share a common mathematical formulation as a dynamical system—a system of several interacting parts whose state evolves continuously with time. The manner in which a dynamical system evolves depends on the form of the interactions. In any neural network the interactions result from the effects one "neuron" has on another by virtue of the connection between them. Thus it is not surprising that the behavior of the neural circuits depends critically on the details of the connections. The particular circuits we have studied have connection patterns appropriate for computing solutions to optimization problems, a class of mathematical problems that involve finding a "best solution" from among a very large number of choices.

The computational behavior exhibited by such circuits is a collective property that results from having many computing elements act on one another in a richly interconnected system. The collective properties can be studied using simplified model neurons, in much the same way as it is possible to understand other large physical systems by greatly reducing the details of their basic components. For example, to study the origin of collective laws of fluid motion, one can simplify the description of complex molecular collisions and produce a tractable model that captures collective features such as temperature and viscosity. Similarly, in seeking to develop a tractable model of the computations carried out by a large number of model neurons, we de-emphasized the details of the processing that goes on at the level of the individual cells and synapses. By simplifying in this way, we were able to discover the general principles by which one can understand collective computation in these circuits.

To comprehend how collective circuits work, it helps to take a very broad view of the essence of computation. Any computing entity, whether it is a digital or analog device or a collection of nerve cells, begins with an initial state and moves through a series of changes to arrive at a state that corresponds to an "answer." The process can be pictured as a path, from initial state to answer, through the physical "configuration space" of the computer as it evolves with time. In a digital computer, for example, the configuration space is defined by the set of voltages for its devices. The input data and program provide initial values for these voltage settings, which change as the computation proceeds and eventually reach a final configuration, which is reported to an output device, such as a screen or a printer.

For any computer there are two critical questions: How does it determine the overall path? And how does it restore itself to that path when physical fluctuations and "noise" cause the computation to drift hopelessly off course (see Figure 10.1)? In a digital computer the path is broken down into logical steps that are embodied in the computer's program. In addition, each computing unit protects against voltage fluctuations by treating a range of voltages, rather than just the exact voltage, as being equal to a nominal value; for example, signals between .8 volt and 1.2 volts can all be restored to 1.0 volt after each logical step in the computation.

In collective-decision circuits the process of computation is significantly different. The overall progress of the computation is determined not by step-by-step instructions but by the rich structure of connections among computing devices. Instead of

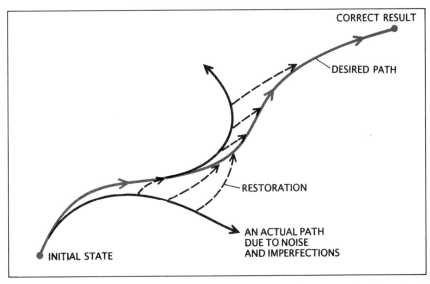

Figure 10.1 COMPUTATIONAL PATH describes how the physical state of a computer changes as it computes. In a digital computer the path is a sequence of discrete steps controlled by the lines of code in a computer program. After each step the computation is restored to the desired path (*red line*). In collective-decision circuits the computational path is continuously focused in a way determined by the pattern of connections in the circuit.

advancing and then restoring the computational path at discrete intervals, the circuit channels or focuses it in one continuous process. These two styles of computation are rather like two different approaches by which a committee makes decisions. In a digital-computer-style committee the members vote yes or no in sequence: each member knows about only a few preceding votes and cannot change a vote once it is cast. In contrast, in a collective-decision committee the members vote together and can express a range of opinions; the members know about all the other votes and can change their opinions. The committee generates a collective decision, or what might be called a sense of the meeting.

The nature of collective computation suggests that it might be particularly effective for problems that involve global interaction between different parts of the problem. We have designed circuits that perform this type of computation to solve certain optimization problems. A typical example is the task-assignment problem, which poses the question: If you have a certain number of assistants and a certain number of tasks, and each assistant does each task at a different rate, how should you assign the tasks so that the corresponding rates add up to

the largest total rate? The neural-network circuit that can solve the problem has many interconnected amplifiers that process the data in parallel. It is able to follow the computational path to a solution rapidly. Because this is a rather complicated circuit, it is helpful to first examine some simple circuits that illuminate the basic principles of all such circuits.

The simplest example for the purpose is the flip-flop, a circuit that is widely used in the electronics industry. The circuit has two stable states—which give it its name—and it makes a decision by choosing one state over the other. It can be built from a pair of saturable amplifiers (see Figure 10.2). In such an amplifier the output voltage increases as the input rises until it reaches a saturation level, beyond which it will not change. The reverse is also true: as the input decreases, the output falls until it saturates at a minimum value. In the flip-flop the output of each of the two amplifiers is inverted (that is, multiplied by −1) and connected to the input of the other. The amplifiers mutually inhibit each other because a high output by either one will drive down the input of the other amplifier. This produces a self-consistent pattern, because each amplifier will drive the other one to be in the opposite state. The

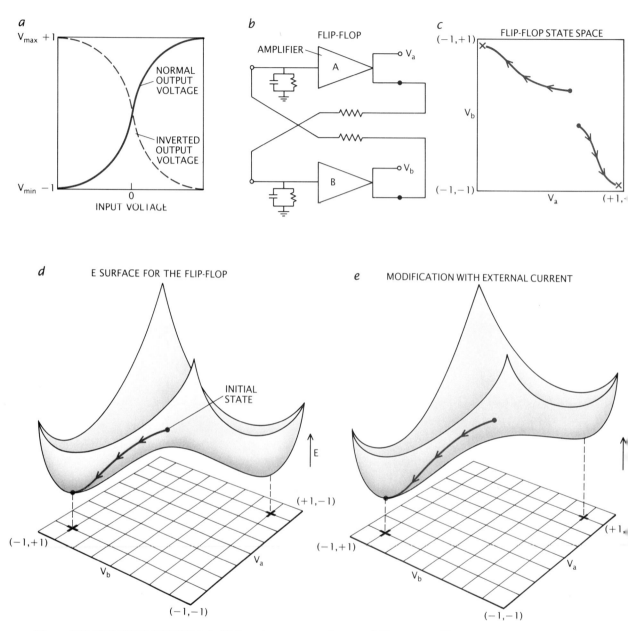

Figure 10.2 FLIP-FLOP CIRCUIT is built from two saturable amplifiers. The output can be normal or inverted (*a*). A resistor connects the output of one amplifier to the input of the other. The normal output terminal (*open circle*) can be used to make an excitatory connection. In the flip-flop the inverted output terminal (*filled circle*) is employed instead to make inhibitory connections. A capacitor and a resistor are connected in parallel at each input to store the charge flowing to the terminal and produce an input voltage and to allow a discharge current to flow (*b*). If the minimum and maximum outputs are + 1 and − 1 and amplifier A is saturated at + 1, B's input will be driven down and B's output will saturate at − 1. The configuration of the amplifier voltages is represented as a point on a two-dimensional plane (*c*). Each axis represents the output of one of the amplifiers, from − 1 to + 1. The circuit will always move to one of the two stable points near (+ 1, − 1) and (− 1, + 1). A third axis represents the value of the computational energy E for each voltage configuration (*d*). The two stable points appear as valleys in the E surface. If an external current is given to one of the amplifiers, this will deepen the valley that corresponds to that amplifier's being in the + 1 state (*e*).

flip-flop therefore has two stable states: if amplifier *A* is putting out +1, then *B* will put out −1, and vice versa. The significant feature of this circuit is that the pattern of the connections is the key to its stability and determines the form of its stable states.

A seemingly remarkable feature of the flip-flop is that no matter what initial inputs are supplied to the circuit when it is turned on, it will make a rapid trajectory to one of the stable states. To understand the phenomenon, picture what happens when a raindrop lands on a terrain of hills and valleys. The drop moves generally downhill until it ends up at the bottom of a nearby valley. The path taken is one in which the gravitational potential energy of the raindrop is continuously decreasing (see Figure 10.3). Similarly, the flip-flop's trajectory is associated with a mathematical quantity we call the computational energy *E*, which can be visualized as a terrain on which the flip-flop's voltage state moves continuously downhill.

E is defined by an explicit mathematical formula that depends on the characteristics of the amplifiers, the strength of the excitatory and inhibitory connections between them, and any external inputs. For

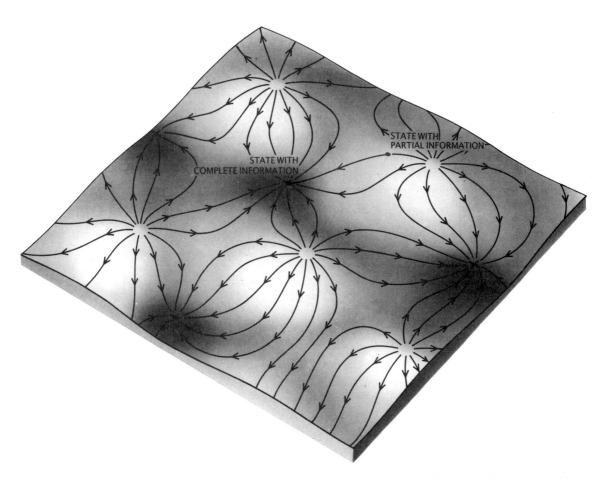

Figure 10.3 COMPUTATIONAL ENERGY of a collective-decision circuit can be pictured as a landscape of hills and valleys. The connection pattern and other physical characteristics of the circuit determine its contours. The circuit computes by following a path that decreases the computational energy until the path reaches the bottom of a valley, just as a raindrop moves downhill to minimize its gravita- tional potential energy. The surface shown here could represent an associative memory, in which the valleys correspond to memories that are stored as associated sets of information (*x*'s). If the circuit is started out with approximate or incomplete information, it follows a path downhill (*colored arrow*) to the nearest valley, which contains the complete information.

fixed inputs in a particular circuit, if E is calculated for each possible configuration of amplifier voltages, it defines a continuous surface. For the flip-flop E can be plotted on a three-dimensional graph (see Figure 10.2). The surface contains two valleys near the voltage configurations $(+1, -1)$ and $(-1, +1)$, which correspond to the two stable states. When the circuit is operating, the changing voltages will describe a downhill motion along the E surface, and eventually the circuit's configuration will come to rest at the bottom of one of the valleys.

The concept of the computational energy proves useful in understanding many features of collective-decision circuits. For example, modifications of the flip-flop circuit alter the shape of the E surface in well-defined ways. If the strengths of the inhibitory connections increase, the valleys become deeper in relation to the "neutral point," or saddle point, in the middle of the E surface. External sources of current also alter the contours of the surface; if a positive current is supplied to the input of one of the amplifiers, it will tend to drive the amplifier to the $+1$ output state. The valley corresponding to this stable configuration will become deeper, and the change will be accompanied by an increase in the size of the "basin of attraction," the area within which any starting point will settle into the stable state at the bottom of the basin. If the external current is large enough, the basin of attraction will fill the entire flip-flop space, eliminating the valley corresponding to the other stable state and leaving only one stable state for the circuit.

The simple flip-flop circuit illustrates how the process of following the trajectory can be interpreted as a process of decision making. For example, the circuit can decide which of two numbers is larger if the amplifiers are given two external input currents that are proportional to the numbers. The amplifier with the larger input will then have a deeper valley at the stable state for which its output is $+1$, and its basin of attraction would expand to include the "neutral point." When the computation is begun by setting the voltages at this point, the circuit state would follow a downhill path to the deeper valley. When the circuit stabilizes, one can note which of the two amplifiers is in the $+1$ state and so determine which number is the larger. For any pair of numbers the corresponding input currents will cause the E surface to change in an appropriate way, thereby ensuring that the path will lead to the correct answer.

For more complicated collective-decision circuits the corresponding E surface acquires so many dimensions that it becomes impossible to draw. Nonetheless, one can understand the general features of the surface and use these as a guide to designing and understanding the circuits. For example, we can generalize from the E surface of the flip-flop to devise a collective-decision circuit that can solve the slightly more difficult problem of determining the largest number in a set of n numbers. The circuit can be thought of as an n-flop, consisting of n amplifiers, each of which is connected to all others with inhibitory connections of equal value. It would have n stable states and its E surface would have n valleys. When a set of input currents is supplied to its amplifiers, the deepest valley would develop for the state that has a $+1$ output for the amplifier receiving the largest input.

In both the flip-flop and the n-flop there is a one-to-one relation between the number of amplifiers and the possible solutions, so that as the number of solutions gets larger, the size of the circuit does too. Is it possible to design a collective circuit that can represent a greater number of solutions than there are amplifiers? Such circuits do indeed exist. They have stable states that consist of configurations of amplifiers in the $+1$ state. This is a more economical use of amplifiers, just as the Roman alphabet is more economical than Chinese ideographs in its use of symbols to encode words.

In 1984 we discovered that networks of this type could rapidly compute good solutions to optimization problems such as the task-assignment problem mentioned above. As an example, imagine you are supervising the job of reshelving books for a large library. You have a number of assistants to do this for you. Each one is familiar with each collection—history, physics and so on—but to varying degrees. Thus Jessica can shelve six books per minute in geology, four per minute in physics and so on, whereas George can shelve one book per minute in geology, eight per minute in physics and so on. You must assign one category to each assistant. How should you assign the tasks so that the total rate of reshelving the books is as high as possible?

One could attack the problem by brute force, trying out every possible combination in sequence. But if there are many assistants and collections, one would soon be overwhelmed by the number of possibilities. If there are n categories of books and n assistants, the number of possible solutions would be the factorial of *n*, or $n(n-1)(n-2) \ldots 1$. There are better iterative digital-computer algorithms that can arrive at an answer in a time period proportional to *n* cubed. The computation could be done even faster, however, if one could take full advantage of the problem's essence: the fact that the proper assignment of each worker depends on the capabilities of every other worker. Ideally the mutual dependencies should be considered simultaneously. It is precisely this kind of computation that can be done quickly and efficiently by a collective-decision circuit.

The data in the task-assignment problem consist of the set of shelving rates. These data can be arranged in a table, in which each row contains the rates for an individual assistant and each column represents a book category (see Figure 10.4). An assignment of tasks can then be thought of as the choice of *n* elements in the table, with the constraint that there can be one and only one element chosen in each row and column, because only one assistant can be assigned to each category. The best solution has the highest sum of rates for the chosen assistants.

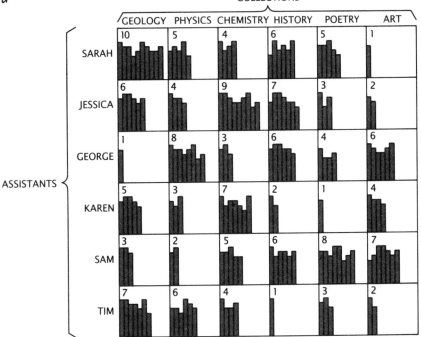

Figure 10.4 TASK-ASSIGNMENT PROBLEM requires assigning each assistant to one collection of books. The rates at which books are shelved per minute are represented in a table (*a*). For this six-by-six problem there are 720 ways to assign the tasks. The pink squares show two possibilities (*b*). The best assignment has the largest sum of shelving rates.

We solved the problem by building an *n*-by-*n* array of amplifiers in which each row corresponds to an assistant and each amplifier in the row corresponds to a different task. The amplifiers in each row and column are linked by mutually inhibitory connections; this provides the constraint that only one assistant can be assigned to each collection, because if one of the amplifiers has a +1 output, the other amplifiers are inhibited. Another way of looking at the circuit is that each row and column is an *n*-flop. These *n*-flops cannot function independently, however, because each amplifier belongs to two such *n*-flops. As you will see below, this pattern of connections is the key to the circuit: it ensures that the circuit will have self-consistent stable states that correspond to possible solutions to the problem (see Figure 10.5).

What are the stable states of this network and what does its *E* surface look like? The stable states consist of configurations of 36 amplifiers in which there are six amplifiers with +1 outputs, with one and only one such amplifier in any row or column.

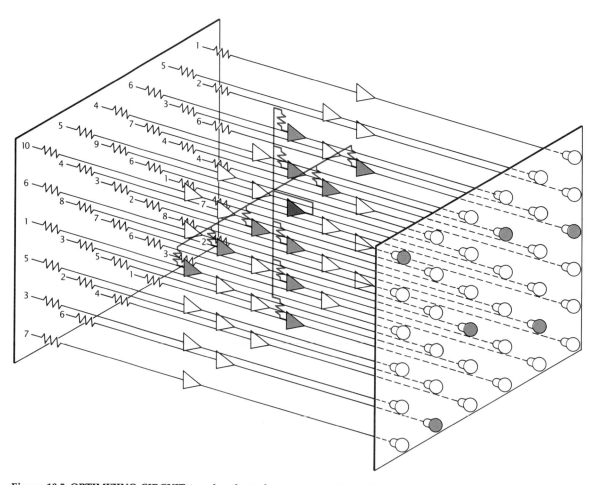

Figure 10.5 OPTIMIZING CIRCUIT to solve the task-assignment problem consists of a network of interconnected *n*-flops. The amplifiers in each row and column are linked by inhibitory connections, which provide the constraint that only one amplifier in any given row and column can be in the +1 state. Because each of the 36 amplifiers in this network inhibits 10 other amplifiers, there are 360 connections altogether. The diagram depicts the connections for one of the amplifiers. The amplifiers receive input currents proportional to the shelving rates. The amplifiers that correspond to the best solution—the combination of inputs that add up to the largest sum—put out a +1 and the rest put out a 0. The +1 outputs can drive a display, such as a light-bulb array.

In a six-by-six array the number of these stable states is 720, or 6 factorial. The E surface for the circuit has valleys of equal depth for each of the 720 possibilities. An input current proportional to the shelving rate of each assistant for each collection is fed to the corresponding amplifier. The valley for each possible solution becomes deeper by an amount proportional to the sum of its corresponding shelving rates.

The network carries out the computation by following a trajectory down the E surface. In the final configuration the circuit usually settles into the deepest valley, which is the correct choice because it corresponds to the task assignment that has the highest total shelving rate. In simulation studies we have shown that this particular circuit will almost always find the best solution to the problem, and a slightly more complex circuit will always find the best solution.

One reason we are interested in studying this type of circuit is that perceptual problems can often be expressed as an optimization. Our senses gather a large set of information about the external world —information that is inevitably imprecise and "noisy." The edge of an object might be hidden behind another object, for example. We know, however, that the edges of objects are continuous, and just because we cannot see an edge does not make us wonder whether the object has changed its shape. Our interpretation of the information is constrained by what we already know.

This knowledge can often be represented as a set of constraints, similar to those in the task-assignment problem, and express it in an E function. The perceptual problem then becomes equivalent to finding the deepest valley in the E surface. For example, Cristof Koch, Jose Marroquin and Alan Yuille, working at the Massachusetts Institute of Technology, showed how several important problems in computer vision could be cast as an optimization problem and solved by a collective-decision circuit in which knowledge of the real world had been imposed as a set of constraints. Their circuit was able to take incomplete depth information of a three-dimensional world and reconstruct missing information such as the locations of the edges of objects.

Another particularly interesting application for collective-decision circuits is associative memory, which is a form of optimization problem. An associative memory is different in principle from a digital-computer memory. A conventional computer stores information by assigning addresses, which identify the physical locations where the data will be stored in hardware, such as a sector or track on a floppy disk. When the central processor requires a piece of data, it issues an instruction to read the data at a particular address. The address itself contains no information about the nature of the data stored there.

Now reflect for a moment about your own memories. If you think of a particular friend, you will remember many facts—name, age, hair color, height, job, hobbies, schooling, family, house, shared experiences and so forth. These facts are somehow combined to form your memory of the individual. There is no notion of storage address in the way you retrieve such information from your memory. Instead pieces of the information itself are used in place of an address.

Associative memory is an idea that came from psychology, not electrical engineering. Fruit flies and garden slugs have associative memories. Indeed, the fact that such relatively simple nervous systems display the phenomenon suggests that it must be a natural—almost spontaneous—property of neuron ensembles. It seems reasonable to ask whether associative memory could also be achieved in networks of artificial neuronlike devices. In the 1970's a number of investigators, including James A. Anderson of Brown University and Teuvo Kohonen of the University of Helsinki, developed mathematical models of associative memory. The concept of the E surface provides a means to understand and study associative-memory circuits built of saturable amplifiers.

How would one make a collective-decision circuit behave like an associative memory? Consider a space of many Cartesian coordinates in which each axis is labeled with some attribute a person might have. One axis might refer to height, one to hair color, one to weight, one to sailing experience, one to the first name of the individual, one to city of residence and so on. Any point in the space describes the characteristics of a hypothetical possible individual. Each of your friends is represented by a particular point in the space. Because you have very few friends compared with the set of all possible individuals, if you put a mark at the position of each of the people you know, you will have marked a very few points in a large space. When someone gives you partial information about a person—for example color of hair and weight but not name—

this describes an approximate location in the space of possible people. The idea of an associative memory is to find the friend who best matches the partial data.

A collective-decision circuit such as the one described for the task-assignment problem could perform as an associative memory if the E surface can be shaped to have valleys, or stable points, at the places that correspond to particular memories. A pattern of input voltages corresponding to a partial memory would be supplied to the amplifiers and the circuit would then follow a trajectory to the bottom of a local valley in the E terrain and read out the output state of the amplifiers as the stored memory. Unlike the task-assignment circuit, in which the connections are highly regular because of the simple global rules that constrain the problem, in an associative memory the connections are irregular and the stable points are scattered somewhat at random because the memories need not have any particular relationship among themselves. To construct an associative memory, therefore, one must find connections between amplifiers such that the many desired memories are represented simultaneously by the circuit's stable states.

A simple associative memory of six interconnected amplifiers illustrates how information can be stored in such a network (see Figure 10.6). The memory states of the system could be described as six-bit binary words, in which each bit corresponds to one of the two possible saturated output states of an amplifier, $+1$ and -1. For example, memory A is $(+1, +1, +1, -1, -1, -1)$. As with the flip-flop circuit, a state can be stable only if it is self-consistent. This is accomplished by ensuring that each amplifier with a $+1$ output has an excitatory connection to the input of every other amplifier that has a $+1$ output and an inhibitory connection to the input of each amplifier that has a -1 output, and vice versa for amplifiers that have -1 outputs. All the inputs to an amplifier are added up to give a big signal with the correct sign. If one looks at the E surface for this associative memory, one will find that the connections have created a valley at the location of the memory.

Because the data are distributed in the pattern of the connections in the circuit, many other memories can be overlaid in the same circuit. It is merely necessary to calculate the connections separately for each memory and add them to the connections for the memories already in storage. This simple additive rule works quite effectively as long as not too many of the same connections are shared among many memories. Problems arise if memories are too similar or too numerous; the valleys on the E surface get too close and begin to interact. (The number of unrelated memories that can be stored effectively is about 15 percent of the number of "neurons" in the circuit.) There are cleverer schemes that can store a larger number of memories or memories that are more similar.

The associative memory described above requires only local information about two linked "neurons" in order to modify the strength of the existing connection between them. This is appealing because it offers a theory of associative memory that is consistent with a biological model proposed more than 30 years ago by Donald O. Hebb. Hebb postulated that biological associative memory must reside in the synaptic connections between nerve cells and that the process of learning and memory storage involves changes in the strength with which nerve signals are transmitted across individual synapses. According to his theory, synapses linking pairs of neurons that are simultaneously active become stronger, thereby reinforcing those pathways in the brain that are excited by specific experiences. As in our associative-memory model, this involves local instead of global changes in the connections. The Hebbian synapse had long eluded actual observation, but recently several investigators have reported evidence for such mechanisms in the brain.

Many laboratories are now exploring how to fabricate and use devices for collective computation. A variety of prototypes have already been built with microelectronic and optical hardware. To be useful, circuits will have to be large, with hundreds or thousands of "neurons," and because these may be densely interconnected, the circuits may contain tens of thousands or even millions of connections. In addition, in order to build a general-purpose circuit such as an associative-memory chip one would need a simple method for modifying the connection strengths.

John J. Lambe and his collaborators, working at the Jet Propulsion Laboratory, constructed from integrated-circuit amplifiers the first associative-memory network of the type we have described. The connections between each pair of amplifiers were chosen through a mechanical switch. The network was expanded to contain 32 amplifiers, with microcomputer-controlled transistor switches replacing

FEATURES ASSIGNED TO NODES

	1	2	3	4	5	6
	NAME	HEIGHT	AGE	WEIGHT	HAIR	EYES
−1	SMITH	TALL	OLD	THIN	BROWN	BLUE
+1	JONES	SHORT	YOUNG	FAT	BLOND	BROWN

NODES

MEMORIES		1	2	3	4	5	6
	A	+1	+1	+1	−1	−1	−1
	B	+1	−1	+1	+1	−1	+1
	C	+1	+1	−1	+1	−1	−1

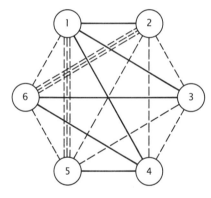 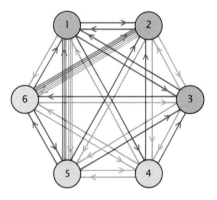

Figure 10.6 ASSOCIATIVE MEMORY with six nodes, or "neurons," is linked by excitatory (*solid line*) and inhibitory (*broken line*) connections. The number of lines in each link represents the strength of the connection; each solid line represents a connection strength of +1, and each broken line represents a strength of −1. Each node might represent a characteristic of a person, as is shown in the table (*a*). Suppose one wants to store three memories, or sets of characteristics (*b*). The nodes that are supposed to be in the +1 state are given an excitatory link to the other +1 nodes and an inhibitory link to the −1 nodes. To store information about all three memories one simply adds up the connections (*c*). For example, the link between nodes 2 and 4 is (−1)+(−1)+(+1), or −1. When the circuit is turned on for memory *A*, the network produces (*d*) the correct pattern of nodes in the +1 state (*red*) and −1 state (*blue*). The pattern is self-consistent: at each node the positive (*red*) and negative (*blue*) incoming currents always add up to have the same sign as the node itself. If the network is given partial data—about a thin, short Jones, for example—it will go into a stable state from which one can retrieve the entire memory.

the mechanical ones. These pioneering circuits work as predicted but are too cumbersome to be of practical use. The first VLSI version was fabricated by Massimo Sivilotti, Michael R. Emreling and Carver A. Mead at the California Institute of Technology (see Figure 10.7). The circuit reduced a 22-amplifier network with 462 interconnections to an area smaller than a square centimeter. The chip functioned as an associative memory when the connection matrix was appropriately programmed. Similar

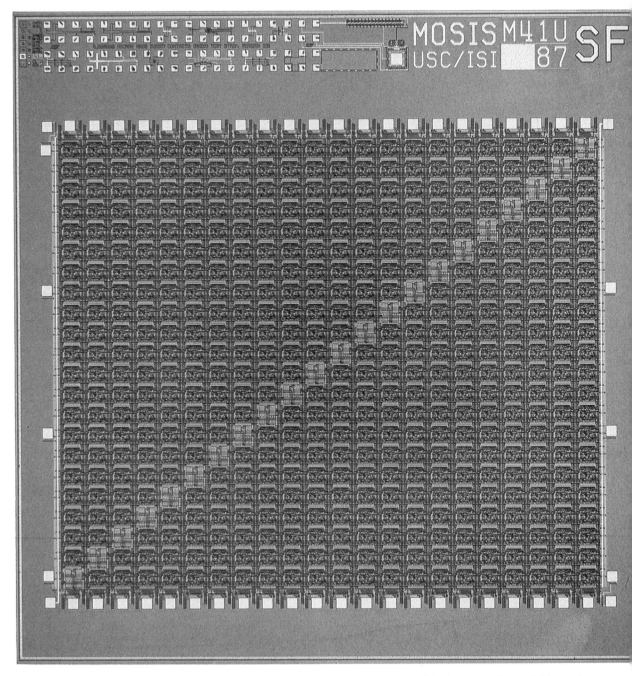

Figure 10.7 VLSI COLLECTIVE-DECISION CIRCUIT was designed in 1985 at the California Institute of Technology by Massimo Sivilotti, Michael R. Emerling and Carver A. Mead. It contains 22 amplifiers, which are the lighter-color components along the diagonal. The devices filling the rest of the square provide the connections, which can be programmed to make the chip an associative memory. The size of the chip is six by six millimeters. (Photo by Melgar Photographers, Inc.)

VLSI circuits with 54 amplifiers have been built by Lawrence D. Jackel, Richard E. Howard and Hans Peter Graf at the AT&T Bell Laboratories. One of the attractive features of collective-decision circuits is that they converge on a good solution rapidly, typically in a few multiples of the characteristic response time of the computing devices. In several of the microelectronic implementations this convergence has occurred in less than one microsecond. Mead's group has recently built a VLSI "artificial retina" chip for image processing, using collective-computation principles in the design.

Advanced optics provides another promising medium for building collective-decision circuits. In that approach light beams would replace the wires. Because light beams can pass through one another without interaction, this raises the possibility of implementing complicated network topologies that might be difficult to achieve in VLSI. Demetri Psaltis and Nabil Farhat have built working prototypes of optical collective circuits [see "Optical Neural Computers," by Yaser S. Abu-Mostafa and Demetri Psaltis; Scientific American, March, 1987].

Many investigators are studying neuronlike circuits different from the ones we have described. A popular model is the feedforward Perceptron, which has been shown to be effective for a broad range of applications, such as pattern recognition. This model consists of simple processing units arranged in several layers. Information is passed into the network through an input layer, and the result of the network's computation is read out at the output layer. There are connections between the layers, and information flows forward only. Such feedforward networks have simplified dynamical behavior and reduced computational capability. On the other hand, many useful learning rules have been devised for such circuits that make it easy to find the appropriate connection pattern. One well-known example, called back-propagation, has been independently derived by David Parker, by David Rumelhart, Geoffrey Hinton and Ronald Williams, and by Paul J. Werbos. One goal of current research is to understand how similar learning algorithms might be applied to networks that have the richer dynamical behavior produced by the kind of feedback employed in the circuits we have discussed.

The study of collective computation in neuronlike circuits has shown that such networks can carry out computations that are not trivial. Computations that are more complicated may require having many simple decisions interact collectively to produce a complex decision. Another feature of many complex decisions is that they must combine information arriving over an extended period of time. Suppose, for example, one wants to identify someone from a distance by the way he walks. One must first make simple decisions about the positions of limbs, combine these over time to determine a sequence of movements and from these form a complex pattern that can be associated with a particular individual. The study of such hierarchical and time-varying collective-decision systems has just begun, but we believe that, as in the case of the circuit-design principles we have described, the research will be propelled by the architectures and design rules of nature's computers.

The Authors

The Editor

RODOLFO R. LLINAS is professor and chairman of the department of physiology and biophysics at the New York University Medical Center in New York. Born in Colombia, he received his M.D. from the Pontifical University of Javeriana in 1959. He then moved to Australia as a research scholar at the Australian National University, from which he received his Ph.D. in 1965, and came to the United States as associate professor at the University of Minnesota. From 1966 to 1970 he was on the staff of the Institute for Biomedical Research of the American Medical Association Education and Research Foundation. In 1970 he became professor of physiology and biophysics and head of the division of neurobiology at the University of Iowa; he left Iowa in 1976 to take up his present job at NYU Medical Center.

HARRY J. JERISON ("Paleoneurology and the Evolution of Mind") is professor of psychiatry and psychology at the University of California School of Medicine in Los Angeles. A native of Poland, he received his Ph.D. from the University of Chicago in 1954. He was a research psychologist at the Aeromedical Laboratory from 1949 until 1957, when he was appointed director of the behavior-research laboratory at Antioch College, a position he held until he moved to UCLA in 1969. Jerison is the author of *Evolution of the Brain and Intelligence* (Academic Press, 1973).

WALLE J. H. NAUTA and **MICHAEL FEIRTAG** ("The Organization of the Brain") have collaborated for more than four years on a textbook of neuroanatomy. Nauta is Institute Professor in the department of psychology at the Massachusetts Institute of Technology and staff neuroanatomist at McLean Hospital in Belmont, Mass. Born in Indonesia, he was educated at the University of Leiden and the University of Utrecht, where he obtained his M.D. in 1942 and his Ph.D. in anatomy and neurophysiology in 1945. He has taught at the universities of Utrecht, Leiden, Zurich and Maryland and he worked as a neurophysiologist at the Walter Reed Army Institute of Research in Washington. In 1964 he joined the MIT faculty. Nauta has received the Research Career Award of the National Institute of Mental Health and the Karl Spencer Lashley Award for research in neurobiology. Feirtag was an editor of *Technology Review*, a magazine published by MIT, at the time this article was written.

W. MAXWELL COWAN ("The Development of the Brain") is vice-president and chief medical scientific officer at the Howard Hughes Medical Institute in Bethesda, Maryland. A native of South Africa, he received his undergraduate education at the University of the Witwatersrand. In 1953 he went to the University of Oxford to obtain his Ph.D. and complete his medical training, and from 1958 until 1966 he was fellow of Pembroke College. In 1966 he emigrated to the U.S. and taught at the University of Wisconsin;

after two years he moved to Washington University. Much of Cowan's scientific work has been on the organization of the limbic system and the development of the visual system.

MARTHA CONSTANTINE-PATON and **MARGARET I. LAW** ("The Development of Maps and Stripes in the Brain") are neurobiologists who share an interest in the development of the visual system. Constantine-Paton is professor of biology at Yale University. Her B.S. is from Tufts University and her Ph.D. from Cornell University. She writes: "I continue to maintain an active interest not only in vision but also in how the auditory and somatosensory systems process information. In fact, I became motivated to study sensory-system development because it seemed that the developmental and functional principles of neural organization might be similar and that a mechanistic understanding of how the brain is put together would help greatly in focusing research aimed at how the mature brain operates." Law has a bachelor's degree from Cornell. She earned her doctorate in 1982 from Princeton for work she did in Constantine-Paton's laboratory on retinotectal specificity.

ARYEH ROUTTENBERG ("The Reward System of the Brain") is professor of psychology and biological sciences and director of the neurosciences program at Northwestern University. He received his bachelor's degree in psychology at McGill University, where he studied physiological psychology with Peter Milner. He then did graduate work at the University of Michigan under James Olds, earning his Ph.D. in 1965. Routtenberg writes: "Olds's intense interest in the biological significance of brain reward convinced me that these neural substrates play a key role in behavior, particularly in memory. As my interest in the anatomical basis of memory has developed I have devoted increasing effort to the study of brain proteins that may participate in memory formation."

MORTIMER MISHKIN and **TIM APPENZELLER** ("The Anatomy of Memory") are respectively chief of the laboratory of neuropsychology at the National Institute of Mental Health (NIMH) and associate editor of SCIENTIFIC AMERICAN. Mishkin has devoted his career to probing the brain mechanisms underlying complex behavior. He is a graduate of Dartmouth College and McGill University, which granted him a Ph.D. in 1951 for work completed at Yale University: an investigation of temporal-lobe function in the primate brain. He then moved to the Institute of Living in Hartford, Conn., where he helped to develop a primate neurobehavioral laboratory; at the same time he commuted to New York University's Bellevue Medical Center to study the effects of brain injuries in wounded war veterans. In 1955 he went to the NIMH to join the section on neuropsychology, a small nucleus of scientists within the laboratory of psychology. Mishkin is past president of the Society for Neuroscience.

NORMAN GESCHWIND ("Specializations of the Human Brain") was James Jackson Putnam Professor of Neurology at the Harvard Medical School, director of the Neurological Unit at Beth Israel Hospital in Boston and professor in the department of psychology and in the School of Health Sciences and Technology at the Massachusetts Institute of Technology. He obtained his bachelor's degree from Harvard College and his M.D. at the Harvard Medical School and then received postgraduate training in Boston and London. Geschwind's research focused on the relation between the anatomy of the brain and behavior, including the cerebral organization of language, aphasias, emotional changes resulting from brain lesions, the evolution of language and the functional asymmetry of the brain. He died in November, 1984.

LYNN A. COOPER and **ROGER N. SHEPARD** ("Turning Something Over in the Mind") are experimental psychologists who have collaborated extensively on the study of mental images. Cooper is professor of psychology at Columbia University, where she runs a computer graphics-based laboratory researching issues in visual cognition and perception. She went to the University of Michigan as an undergraduate and received her Ph.D. from Stanford University in 1973. Cooper has won the American Psychological Association's Distinguished Scientific Award for an Early Career Contribution to Psychology. Shepard is professor of psychology at Stanford University. He earned his undergraduate degree at Stanford in 1951 and his Ph.D. from Yale University in 1955. In 1968 he returned to Stanford as a member of the faculty. He has received the Distinguished Scientific Contribution Award of the American Psychological Association and is a member of the National Academy of Sciences. Shepard and Cooper first worked together when she was a graduate student at Stanford; the book *Mental Images and Their Transformations* (The MIT Press/ Bradford Books, 1982), of which they are coauthors, surveys their ensuing research.

ADRIAN R. MORRISON ("A Window on the Sleeping Brain") is professor of anatomy at the School of Veterinary Medicine at the University of Pennsylvania. He has two degrees from Cornell University: a D.V.M. (1960) and an M.S. (1962). His Ph.D. in anatomy

(1964) is from the University of Pennsylvania. After a year of postdoctoral work at the University of Pisa he returned to Pennsylvania, where he has remained.

DAVID W. TANK and **JOHN J. HOPFIELD** ("Collective Computation in Neuronlike Circuits") work together on the technical staff of the AT&T Bell Laboratories. Tank has a B.S. degree from Case Western Reserve University. He joined Bell Laboratories in 1983, the year he received his Ph.D. in physics from Cornell University. Hopfield has been at Bell Laboratories since 1973 and is also Roscoe Gilkey Dickinson Professor of chemistry and biology at the California Institute of Technology. He received a Ph.D. in physics from Cornell University in 1958 and spent two years at Bell Laboratories before accepting a position as a research physicist at the École Normale Supérieure. He returned to the U.S. in 1961 to teach physics at the University of California at Berkeley, leaving there in 1964 for Princeton University. He took his post at Caltech in 1980.

Bibliographies

1. Paleoneurology and the Evolution of Mind

Uexküll, Jakob von. 1957. A stroll through the worlds of animals and men: A picture book of invisible worlds. In *Instinctive behavior: The development of a modern concept*, ed. and trans. Claire H. Schiller. International Universities Press, Inc.

Eccles, John C. 1970. *Facing reality: Philosophical adventures by a brain scientist.* Springer-Verlag New York, Inc.

Tobias, Phillip V. 1971. *The brain in hominid evolution.* Columbia University Press.

Popper, Karl R. 1972. *Objective knowledge: An evolutionary approach.* Oxford University Press.

Jerison, Harry J. 1973. *Evolution of the brain and intelligence.* Academic Press.

2. The Organization of the Brain

Herrick, C. Judson. 1924. *Neurological foundations of animal behavior.* Henry Holt and Company.

Nauta, Walle J. H., and Harvey J. Karten. 1970. A general profile of the vertebrate brain with sidelights on the ancestry of cerebral cortex. In *The neurosciences: Second study program.* ed. Francis O. Schmitt. Rockefeller University Press.

Warwick, Roger, and Peter L. Williams, eds. 1973. Neurology. In *Gray's Anatomy*, 35th British ed. W. B. Saunders Company.

3. The Development of the Brain

Hunt, R. Kevin. 1975. Developmental programming for retinotectal patterns. In *Cell patterning: Ciba Foundation symposium 29.* Associated Scientific Publishers.

Rakic, P. 1975. Cell migration and neuronal ectopias in the brain. *Birth defects: Original articles series* 11:95–129.

Hubel, D. H., T. N. Wiesel and S. LeVay. 1977. Plasticity of ocular dominance columns in monkey striate cortex. *Philosophical Transactions of the Royal Society of London, Series B* 278 (April 26): 377–409.

Cowan, W. Maxwell. 1978. Aspects of neural development. In *International review of physiology: Neurophysiology III*, ed. R. Porter. University Park Press.

Jacobson, Marcus. 1978. *Developmental neurobiology.* Plenum Press.

4. The Development of Maps and Stripes in the Brain

Sperry, R. W. 1963. Chemoaffinity in the orderly growth of nerve fiber patterns and connections. *Proceedings of the National Academy of Sciences* 50 (October 15): 703–710.

Stent, Gunther S. 1973. A physiological mechanism for Hebb's postulate of learning. *Proceedings of the National Academy of Sciences* 70 (April): 997–1001.

Malsburg, Ch. von der, and W. J. Willshaw. 1976. A mechanism for producing continuous neural mappings: Ocularity dominance stripes and ordered retino-tectal projections. *Experimental Brain Research*, Supplement 1:463–469.

Law, M. I., and M. Constantine-Paton. 1981. Anatomy and physiology of experimentally produced striped tecta. *Journal of Neuroscience* 1 (July): 741–759.

5. The Reward System of the Brain

Lindvall, Olle, and Anders Björklund. 1974. The organization of the ascending catecholamine neuron systems in the rat brain as revealed by the glyoxylic acid fluorescence method. *Acta Physiologica Scandinavica Supplementum* 412:1–48.

Wauquier, Albert, and Edmund T. Rolls. 1976. *Brain stimulation reward.* North-Holland Publishing Company.

Olds, James. 1977. *Drives and reinforcements: Behavioral studies of hypothalamic functions.* Raven Press.

Routtenberg, Aryeh, and Rebecca Santos-Anderson. 1977. The role of prefrontal cortex in intracranial self-stimulation. In *Handbook of psycholopharmacology: Vol. 8*, eds. Leslie L. Iversen, Susan D. Iversen and Solomon H. Snyder. Plenum Press.

6. The Anatomy of Memory

Mishkin, M. 1982. A memory system in the monkey. *Philosophical Transactions of the Royal Society of London*, Series B 298 (June 25): 85–95.

Mishkin, M., Barbara Malamut and Jocelyne Bachevalier. 1984. Memories and habits: Two neural systems. In *Neurobiology of learning and memory*, eds. Gary Lynch, James L. McGaugh and Norman M. Weinberger. The Guilford Press.

Aggleton, John P., and M. Mishkin. 1985. The amygdala: Sensory gateway to the emotions. In *Emotion: Theory, research and experience, vol. 3,* eds. Robert Plutchik and Henry Kellerman. Academic Press.

Murray, Elisabeth A., and M. Mishkin. 1985. Amygdalectomy impairs crossmodal association in monkeys. *Science* 228 (May 3): 604–606.

7. Specializations of the Human Brain

Gainotti, G. 1972. Emotional behavior and hemispheric side of the lesion. *Cortex* 8 (March): 41 55.

Geschwind, Norman. 1974. *Selected papers on language and the brain.* D. Reidel Publishing Company.

Gazzaniga, Michael S., and Joseph E. Ledoux. 1978. *The integrated mind.* Plenum Press.

Galaburda, Albert M., Marjorie LeMay, Thomas L. Kemper and Norman Geschwind. 1978. Right-left asymmetries in the brain. *Science* 199 (February 24): 852–856.

8. Turning Something Over in the Mind

Shepard, R. N., and J. Metzler. 1971. Mental rotation of three-dimensional objects. *Science* 171 (February 19): 701–703.

Cooper, Lynn A. 1975. Mental rotation of random two-dimensional shapes. *Cognitive Psychology* 7 (January): 20–43.

Hochberg, Julian E. 1978. *Perception.* Prentice-Hall, Inc.

Shepard, R. N. 1984. Ecological constraints on internal representation: Resonant kinematics of perceiving, imagining, thinking and dreaming. *Psychological Review* 91 (October): 417–447.

9. A Window on the Sleeping Brain

Drucker-Colin, René, Mario Shkurovich and M. B. Sterman, eds. 1979. *The functions of sleep.* Academic Press, Inc.

Chase, M. H., ed. 1982. *Sleep disorders: Intersections of basic and clinical research.* Spectrum Publications, Inc.

Hendricks, J. C., A. R. Morrison and G. L. Mann. 1982. Different behaviors during paradoxical sleep without atonia depend on pontine lesion site. *Brain Research* 23:81–105.

10. Collective Computation in Neuronlike Circuits

Denker, John, ed. 1986. *Computing with neural networks.* American Institute of Physics.

Rumelhart, David E., James L. McClelland and the PDP Research Group, eds. 1986. *Parallel distributed processing: Explorations in the microstructure of cognition.* The MIT Press.

Hopfield, J. J., and D. W. Tank. 1986. Computing with neural circuits: A model. *Science* 233 (August 8): 625–633.

INDEX

Page numbers in *italics* indicate illustrations.